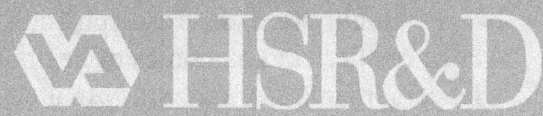

I0488927

Pain in Patients with Polytrauma: A Systematic Review

September 2008

Prepared for:

Department of Veterans Affairs
Veterans Health Administration
Health Services Research & Development Service
Washington, DC 20420

Prepared by:

Portland Veterans Affairs Healthcare System
Oregon Evidence-based Practice Center
Portland, OR

Investigators:

Steven K. Dobscha, MD
Principal Investigator

Rose Campbell, MLIS, MS
Research Associate

Benjamin J. Morasco, PhD
Investigator

Michele Freeman, MPH
Research Associate

Mark Helfand, MD, MPH
Director

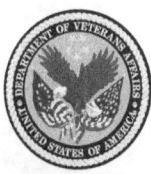

PREFACE

VA's Health Services Research and Development Service (HSR&D) works to improve the cost, quality, and outcomes of health care for our nation's veterans. Collaborating with VA leaders, managers, and policy makers, HSR&D focuses on important health care topics that are likely to have significant impact on quality improvement efforts. One significant collaborative effort is HSR&D's Evidence-based Synthesis Program (ESP). Through this program, HSR&D provides timely and accurate evidence syntheses on targeted health care topics. These products will be disseminated broadly throughout VA and will: inform VA clinical policy, develop clinical practice guidelines, set directions for future research to address gaps in knowledge, identify the evidence to support VA performance measures, and rationalize drug formulary decisions.

HSR&D provided funding for the two Evidence Based Practice Centers (EPCs) supported by the Agency for Healthcare Research and Quality (AHRQ) that also had an active and publicly acknowledged VA affiliation—Southern California EPC and Portland, OR EPC— so they could develop evidence syntheses on requested topics for dissemination to VA policymakers. A planning committee with representation from HSR&D, Patient Care Services, Office of Quality and Performance, and the VISN Clinical Management Officers, has been established to identify priority topics and to ensure the quality of final reports. Comments on this evidence report are welcome and can be sent to Susan Schiffner, ESP Program Manager, at Susan.Schiffner@va.gov.

Pain in Patients with Polytrauma

EXECUTIVE SUMMARY

BACKGROUND

Pain resulting from polytraumatic injuries poses numerous challenges during and after rehabilitation treatment. The objectives of this report are to systematically review the literature to address the assessment and management of pain in patients with polytraumatic injuries, to identify patient, clinician and systems factors associated with pain-related outcomes in these patients, and to describe current or planned research addressing the key questions in this report.

The key questions were:

1. Have reliable and valid measures and assessment tools been developed to measure pain intensity and pain-related functional interference among patients with cognitive deficits due to TBI? Which measures and tools are likely to be most useful in assessing pain in polytrauma patients with cognitive deficits due to TBI?

2. A. Which treatment approaches are most likely to be effective in improving pain outcomes (pain intensity and functional interference) in polytrauma patients?
   B. Which pain treatment approaches are most likely to enhance overall rehabilitation efforts?

3. A. Does blast-related headache pain differ in terms of phenomenology and treatment from other types of headache pain?
   B. Which treatments are best for persistent blast-related headache pain?

4. What patient factors are associated with better and worse pain-related clinical outcomes among polytrauma patients? Have interventions been developed to specifically address these factors?

5. What are unique provider and system barriers to detecting and treating pain among polytrauma patients? Have interventions been developed to effectively address these barriers?

We also sought to identify and describe current or planned research that is addressing or will address the key questions.

METHODS

Literature Search
Two research librarians independently designed search strategies based on the key questions, and conducted searches in Medline of literature published from 1950 through July 2008. The results of both searches were combined into a single reference library. Three researchers trained in the critical analysis of literature assessed for relevance the abstracts of citations identified from these literatures searches. Full-text articles of potentially relevant abstracts were retrieved for further review. Reference lists from

articles were reviewed to find additional articles for inclusion. We also searched for in-progress and unpublished trials. Due to a limited number of studies using controls or comparators, we included cross-sectional and case report/case series studies in the review for some key questions, We systematically rated the quality of cohort and case-control design studies.

Active Research

The PI sent email communications inquiring about active or planned research to a number of groups and individuals identified through VA workgroups, personal knowledge of investigators, recent publications, and several web-databases which included information about funded VA and non-VA projects. Email communications described the evidence review project, and asked respondents to describe any relevant projects they were involved in or planning as well as to identify other investigators who might be working in these areas (snowball approach). Initial email messages were sent at the end of January 2008; email messages to newly identified investigators and follow-up communications occurred continuously until August 28, 2008.

RESULTS

We screened 3252 titles and performed a more detailed review of 578 articles. From these, we identified one systematic review, one qualitative research study, and 93 observational studies that addressed at least one of the key questions. Studies were excluded for the following reasons: 1) the study population did not constitute or include polytrauma patients or patients with blast-related headaches; 2) the study addressed perioperative or surgical pain management or management of specific orthopedic injuries or only short term (less than 3 months post-injury) outcomes; 3) the study outcomes did not include measures of pain intensity or pain-related function; 4) the text of the article was non-English. The primary findings for each key question are summarized below. Secondary findings are presented in further detail within the report.

KEY QUESTION #1 Have reliable and valid measures and assessment tools been developed to measure pain intensity and pain-related functional interference among patients with cognitive deficits due to TBI? Which measures and tools are likely to be most useful in assessing pain in polytrauma patients with cognitive deficits due to TBI?

There were no published studies that assessed measures of pain intensity or pain-related functional interference among patients with cognitive deficits due to TBI.

KEY QUESTION #2 A. Which treatment approaches are most likely to be effective in improving pain outcomes (pain intensity and functional interference) in polytrauma patients? B. Which pain treatment approaches are most likely to enhance overall rehabilitation efforts?

2A: There were no randomized controlled trials, systematic reviews, prospective cohort, case-control, or systematic observational studies that tested the efficacy or effectiveness of specific pain treatment approaches among patients with polytrauma.

2B: One fair-quality retrospective cohort study of patients with trauma-related amputation demonstrated that after controlling for demographic factors, injury characteristics and other medical morbidity, inpatient rehabilitation was marginally associated with increased likelihood of return to work and decreased likelihood of reduced hours of work.(GRADE: Very Low)

KEY QUESTION #3 A. Does blast-related headache pain differ in terms of phenomenology and treatment from other types of headache pain? B. Which treatments are best for persistent blast-related headache pain?

There were no randomized controlled trials, cohort studies, case-control studies, or other systematic observational studies that compared patients with blast-related headache to patients with other types of headache or that specifically addressed treatments for blast-related related headache pain.

KEY QUESTION #4 What patient factors are associated with better and worse clinical outcomes among polytrauma patients? Have interventions been developed to specifically address these factors?

There were no randomized controlled trials. One systematic review, 9 cohort, 3 case-control, and 13 cross-sectional studies specifically addressed patient factors associated with outcomes in TBI patients. Thirty-two cohort, 11 cross-sectional, and 4 case-control studies addressed patient factors associated with outcomes in patients with other types of polytraumatic injuries.

Traumatic Brain Injury
   One fair-quality systematic review involving 23 studies and 4,206 patients showed that overall, 58% of patients with TBI have chronic headache, and that brain injury is associated with headache even after adjustment for post-traumatic stress disorder (PTSD). This review also found that patients with mild TBI were more likely to have headache than patients with moderate or severe TBI. However, our review, which included studies not included in the above study, showed mixed findings regarding the association between severity of TBI and pain (GRADE: Very Low).

   Psychological factors, including depression and posttraumatic stress disorder (PTSD), and insomnia and fatigue are associated with pain in TBI patients. (GRADE: Low)

Other injuries in polytrauma patients
   Characteristics of injuries (location, severity, and whether they are multiple) are associated with clinical outcomes including persistent pain and functional status. Specific factors associated with worse pain-related outcomes include: multiple injuries,

foot injuries or injuries below the knee joint, and concurrent head injury or cognitive disability. (GRADE: Low)

Other factors associated with better outcomes in some studies of patients with polytraumatic injuries other than TBI were younger age, higher educational achievement, having a white collar job or higher income. (GRADE: Very Low)

KEY QUESTION #5 What are unique provider and system barriers to detecting and treating pain among polytrauma patients? Have interventions been developed to effectively address these barriers?

There were no randomized controlled trials, cohort studies, case-control studies, or other systematic observational studies that addressed provider and system barriers to detecting and treating pain among polytrauma patients. One qualitative study of providers from four VA Polytrauma Rehabilitation Centers (PRCs) addressed potential provider and system barriers to treating polytrauma patients. In interviews, providers reported that polytrauma patients are very complex to treat, and that the work with this population is very challenging and emotionally taxing. The investigators and study respondents suggested that increasing use of multidisciplinary and concurrent care and consultation from experts may be necessary to provide the care that is needed.

Results—Active Research

Nineteen relevant active or planned projects were identified and project data were collected on 18 of these projects. Fifteen of the studies should generate information regarding patient factors that may contribute to pain-related outcomes among polytrauma patients (Key Question 4), and 4 studies are testing interventions for pain among polytrauma patients (Key Question 2). One active study will test the reliability and validity of measures to assess pain in cognitively-impaired TBI patients and another study is using primarily qualitative methods to examine the utility of a Computerized Patient Record System (CPRS) pain assessment template module to assist clinicians in evaluating pain in PRC patients with cognitive impairment (Key Question 1). One study is examining the phenomenology and treatment of blast vs. other types of headache (Key Question 3), and one study is addressing provider and systems barriers to detecting and treating pain in polytrauma patients (Key Question 5).

Pain in Patients with Polytrauma

TABLE OF CONTENTS

Pain in Patients with Polytrauma

Pain in Patients with Polytrauma

INTRODUCTION

Polytrauma is defined in the VHA Polytrauma Rehabilitation Centers Directive dated June 8, 2005 as: "injury to the brain in addition to other body parts or systems resulting in physical, cognitive, psychological, or psychosocial impairments and functional disability." The definition of polytrauma has since expanded to include concurrent injury to two or more body parts or systems that results in cognitive, physical, psychological or other psychosocial impairments. Traumatic Brain Injury (TBI) often occurs in polytrauma and in combination with other disabling conditions including amputation, auditory or visual impairments, spinal cord injury (SCI), post-traumatic stress disorder (PTSD), and other mental health conditions.

Pain resulting from polytraumatic injuries poses numerous challenges during rehabilitation treatment and afterwards. Treatments typically used to reduce pain in these individuals (for example, oral opioids) have the potential to interfere with the active rehabilitation needed to restore function.

The objectives of this report are to systematically review the literature to address the assessment and management of pain in patients with polytraumatic injuries, to identify patient, clinician and systems factors associated with pain-related outcomes in these patients, and to describe current or planned research addressing the key questions.

Background

Major advances in body armor technology and battlefield medicine have improved survival from combat injuries that would have been fatal in previous wars.(1) Data from the Department of Defense indicate that the lethality of war wounds has decreased from 24% in the Vietnam and Persian Gulf Wars to 10% in the current Operation Enduring Freedom/Operation Iraqi Freedom (OEF/OIF) conflicts.(2) Survivors of polytraumatic injuries among soldiers returning from the current conflicts tend to have more complex injuries and emotional trauma than typically seen in the past wars.(3, 4)

Among 119 casualties admitted to Walter Reed Army Medical Center from OIF during March 1 to July 1, 2003, 39% had sustained gunshot wounds, 31% sustained blast and shrapnel injuries, and 34% had blunt/motor vehicle collision mechanisms.(5) Among these 119 patients there were 184 injured areas, and the location of injury was the lower extremity for 62% of patients, the upper extremity for 30%, the head and neck for 25%, the chest for 25%, and the abdomen for 16%. Among 52 patients with orthopedic injuries evacuated during OEF between December 2001 and January 2003, 15 (29%) had suffered traumatic amputations, of which 5 (33.3%) were below-knee.(6) All amputations were caused by land mines or exploded ordinance.

Twenty-eight percent of all individuals medically evacuated to the Walter Reed Army Medical Center (WRAMC) due to combat injuries during OEF/OIF had a TBI, according to a report in 2006.(4) By contrast, 12 to 14% of all combat casualties in the Vietnam War had a brain injury.(7) In the current conflicts, Kevlar body armor and helmets have improved overall survival rates and reduced the frequency of penetrating head injuries.(7) Because mortality from substantial brain injuries among U.S. combatants in Vietnam was 75% or greater, soldiers with recognized brain injuries made up only a small fraction of the casualties. Between January 2003 and February 2005, 59% of all patients who were exposed to a blast and admitted to WRAMC were given a diagnosis of TBI.(7) Closed TBI accounted for 88% of all TBI. Moderate to severe TBI accounted for 56% of TBI cases. Nineteen percent of TBI patients sustained concomitant amputation.

Brain injuries from blasts may go undiagnosed and untreated in patients with polytrauma because of the attention focused on more visible injuries. Commonly overlooked pain-related conditions in patients with polytrauma may include soft-tissue damage, PTSD, nerve damage, hearing loss and tinnitus, chronic infections, vision changes, lung injury, vestibular problems, and undiscovered shrapnel fragments.(8) In addition to the direct effects of blasts, injuries can result from the structural collapse and fragmentation of buildings and vehicles, and may include crush injuries and compartment syndrome.(9)

Under a new system established by the VHA in 2005, severely injured soldiers with TBI are being referred early in their treatment to one of four VA medical centers in Richmond, VA; Tampa, FL; Palo Alto, CA; and Minneapolis, MN) designated as Polytrauma Rehabilitation Centers (PRCs). The four PRCs approach treatment of polytrauma patients using a mechanism-of-injury approach to provide a comprehensive, efficient, and interdisciplinary system of care.(8) Each of the four PRCs has been identifying six to 10 cases of TBI per month that were missed in military hospitals.(10)

METHODS

Topic Development

This topic was nominated by Michael Clark, PhD, Clinical Director of the Pain Program, James A. Haley VAMC. The scope and key questions for the review were further refined in consultation with representatives from the VA HSR&D Service, the VA Evidence Synthesis Program, and technical experts in pain, polytrauma, or traumatic brain injury (Robert Kerns, PhD; Nina Sayer, PhD; Marti Buffum DNSc, APRN, BC, CS; Michael Clark, PhD; Henry Lew, MD, PhD; Nancy Carney, PhD; Ron Gironda, PhD; Martin Schreiber, MD).

1. Have reliable and valid measures and assessment tools been developed to measure pain intensity and pain-related functional interference among patients with cognitive deficits due to TBI? Which measures and tools are likely to be most useful in assessing pain in polytrauma patients with cognitive deficits due to TBI?

2. A. Which treatment approaches are most likely to be effective in improving pain outcomes (pain intensity and functional interference) in polytrauma patients?
   B. Which pain treatment approaches are most likely to enhance overall rehabilitation efforts?

3. A. Does blast-related headache pain differ in terms of phenomenology and treatment from other types of headache pain?
   B. Which treatments are best for persistent blast-related headache pain?

4. What patient factors are associated with better and worse pain-related clinical outcomes among polytrauma patients? Have interventions been developed to specifically address these factors?

5. What are unique provider and system barriers to detecting and treating pain among polytrauma patients? Have interventions been developed to effectively address these barriers?

Polytrauma is defined as concurrent injury to two or more body parts or systems resulting in cognitive, physical, psychological or other psychosocial impairments. Combat-related mental conditions co-occurring with injury to at least one other system also constitutes polytrauma.

The scope of this review **includes** the assessment and treatment in rehabilitation and post-rehabilitation care settings of persistent pain or exacerbations of pain resulting from polytraumatic injuries. We included studies measuring pain-related outcomes, specifically pain intensity and pain-related function or interference, 3 months or more from the date of injury.

The scope of this review **excludes** the following:
- Short-term (less than 3 months) outcomes following injury. We sought to focus on pain persisting into the rehabilitation phase of treatment or longer, and not battlefield or acute management of polytraumatic injury.
- Unilateral amputation without other concurrent conditions or injuries. Bilateral amputation was considered polytrauma.
- Spinal cord injury without other concurrent conditions or injuries
- Choice of specific surgical strategy or specific procedures for particular orthopedic injuries or perioperative management of traumatic injuries.
- Post-traumatic/post-concussive headache unrelated to blast injury, unless the sample includes patients with moderate or greater TBI.
- Functional outcomes of polytrauma unless pain measures are included as one component of the functional outcome measure or in addition to the functional outcome measure.

Figure 1 illustrates the analytic framework that guided our review and synthesis.

Pain in Patients with Polytrauma

Figure 1. Analytic Framework

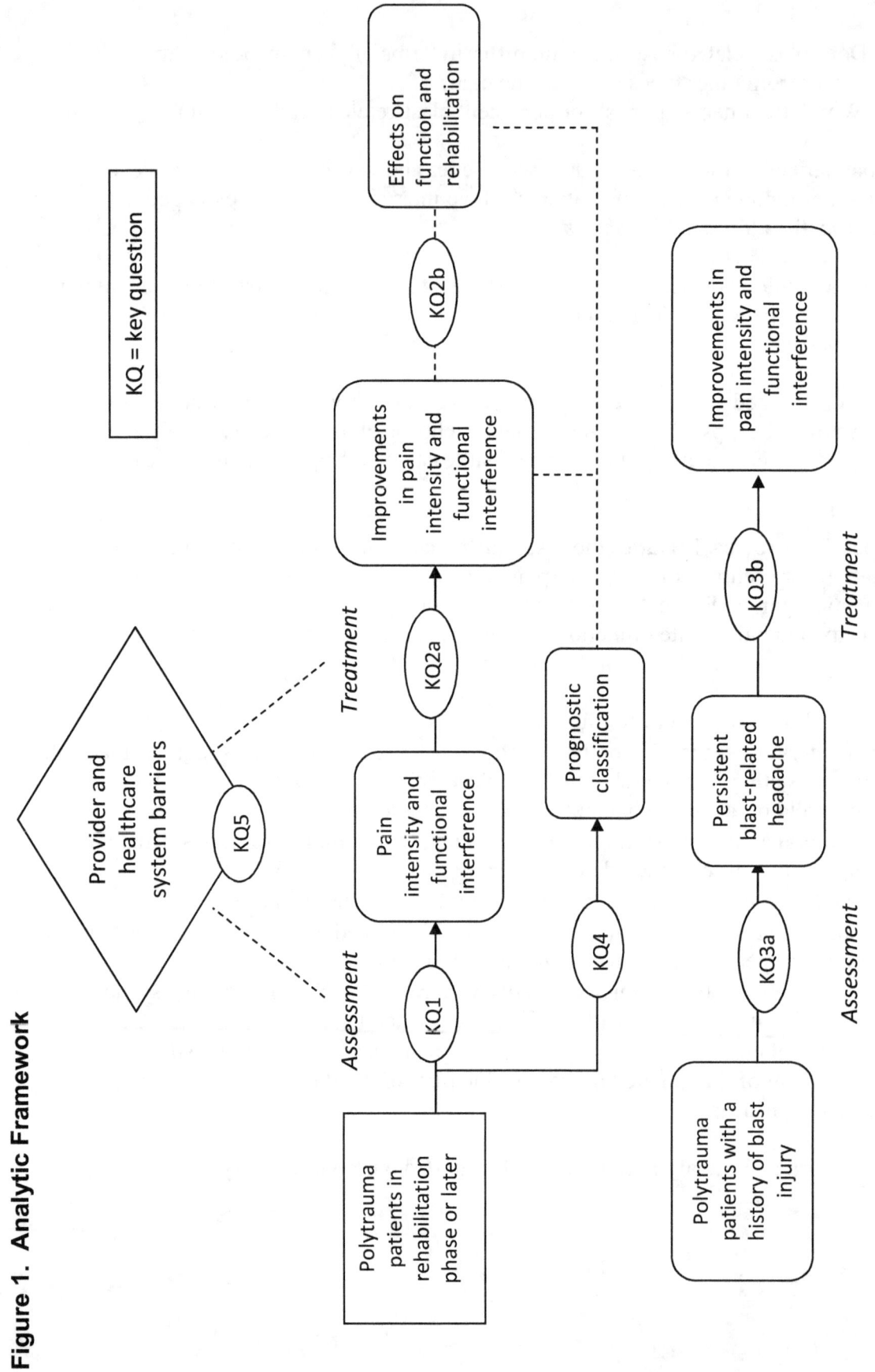

Literature Search Strategy

Two research librarians (Rose Campbell and Andrew Hamilton) independently designed search strategies based on the key questions, and conducted searches in Medline of literature published from 1950 through July 2008. Appendix A provides the search strategies in detail. The results of both searches were combined into a single reference library. Additional articles were identified from reference lists of studies, review articles, editorials, and by consulting experts. We also searched for relevant studies in the following databases: PsychINFO; the PILOTS Database (the VA PTSD bibliographic database); REHABDATA, the bibliographic database of the National Rehabilitation Information Center; the DoD Defense Technical Information Center; and the Cochrane Database of controlled clinical trials. All citations were imported into an electronic database (EndNote X1). We also searched for unpublished and ongoing research studies, as described in the section on Active Research to follow.

Study Selection

Three researchers (SD, RC, MF) trained in the critical analysis of literature reviewed the titles and abstracts identified from the searches. Full-text articles of potentially relevant abstracts were retrieved for further review. Each article retrieved was reviewed with a brief screening form (see Appendix B) that collected data on the key question to which the article applied, as well as key words or emerging themes. Reference lists from pertinent articles were reviewed to find additional articles for inclusion.

Study Inclusion Criteria

Eligible articles had English-language abstracts and provided primary data relevant to the key questions. For a study to be eligible for Key Questions 1, 2, 4 and 5, the sample had to have all or a majority of patients with polytrauma, or analyses and findings had to be stratified by whether the patients had polytrauma, such that if a minority of the sample had polytrauma, readers could discern outcomes for the polytrauma group. For purposes of the review, polytrauma was defined as concurrent injury to two or more body parts or systems resulting in cognitive, physical, psychological or other psychosocial impairments. TBI of moderate or greater severity was also considered polytrauma (head injury itself plus associated cognitive sequellae). Combat-related mental conditions co-occurring with injury to at least one other system also constituted polytrauma. This definition is consistent with the VHA Directive 2005-024 describing the policy for the PRCs. Eligible studies examined the assessment and treatment in rehabilitation and post-rehabilitation care settings of persistent pain or exacerbations of pain resulting from polytraumatic injuries.

Eligible study designs included controlled clinical trials, systematic reviews, as well as prospective and retrospective cohort studies, case-control design studies, and qualitative studies using rigorous qualitative research methods. For these types of study designs, we abstracted data as described below. Due to a limited number of studies that included a comparator group, we also considered relevant cross-sectional and case report/case series studies for inclusion for some of the key questions. For these study designs, data were not formally abstracted nor rated for quality of evidence.

Study Exclusion Criteria

Studies examining battlefield/emergency or assessment and care within 3 months of injury were not included unless they also examined pain outcomes 3 months or more from the date of injury, that is, pain persisting into the rehabilitation phase of treatment or longer. We also did not include studies examining choice of specific surgical strategy, the perioperative management of traumatic injuries (including burn injuries), or use of particular procedures or devices for specific orthopedic injuries. There are numerous case reports and case series describing specific surgical interventions for particular types of wounds; we felt that their inclusion would not yield generalizable information. We excluded studies describing functional outcomes of polytrauma unless a pain measure was included and reported as a component of the functional outcome measure or in addition to the functional outcome measure. Finally, we excluded studies of post-traumatic/post-concussive headache unless the sample included patients with moderate or more severe head injury or included a majority of patients with blast-related head injury. There have been a number of narrative reviews of assessment and treatment of post-traumatic headache among patients with mild-TBI or post-concussive syndrome; we felt that inclusion of these studies was beyond the scope of our key questions.

Secondary Findings

For key questions 1, 2, 3, and 4, the investigators included additional information (labeled *Secondary Findings*) from studies that were formally excluded during the search and abstraction process, but which contained information that seemed pertinent to the key questions and which we felt may be of interest to readers. This additional information does not reflect results of a comprehensive, systematic literature search on the specific secondary findings topics; rather it reflects information derived from manuscripts identified during our main search process.

Data Abstraction

We abstracted the following data from included studies: study design, setting, objectives, eligibility criteria, sample size, intervention or exposure of interest, comparator intervention or control group, outcomes measured, timing of outcome assessment, years of enrollment/observation, duration of follow-up, demographics, potential confounders considered, results, and conclusions.

Quality Assessment

We assessed the quality of studies when applicable, using criteria developed by the US Preventive Services Task Force(11) for rating randomized controlled trials, cohort studies, and case control studies (Appendix C). We did not rate the quality of cross-sectional studies, case reports, or case series.

Data Synthesis

We constructed evidence tables showing the study characteristics and results for all included studies, organized by key question, intervention, or clinical condition, as appropriate. We critically analyzed studies to compare their characteristics, methods, and findings. We compiled a summary of findings for each key question or clinical topic, and drew conclusions based on qualitative synthesis of the findings.

Rating the body of evidence

We assessed the overall quality of evidence for outcomes using a method developed by the Grading of Recommendations, Assessment, Development, and Evaluation (GRADE) Working Group, which classified the grade of evidence across outcomes according to the following criteria:(12)

High = Further research is very unlikely to change our confidence on the estimate of effect.
Moderate = Further research is likely to have an important impact on our confidence in the estimate of effect and may change the estimate.
Low = Further research is very likely to have an important impact on our confidence in the estimate of effect and is likely to change the estimate.
Very Low = Any estimate of effect is very uncertain.

The GRADE Working Group also suggests using the following scheme for assigning the "grade" or strength of evidence:

Criteria for assigning GRADE of evidence

Type of evidence
Randomized trial = high
Observational study = low
Any other evidence = very low

Decrease GRADE if:
- Serious (-1) or very serious (-2) limitation to study quality
- Important inconsistency (-1)
- Some (-1) or major (-2) uncertainty about directness
- Imprecise or sparse data (-1)
- High probability of reporting bias (-1)

Increase GRADE if:
- Strong evidence of association-significant relative risk of >2 (<0.5) based on consistent evidence from two or more observational studies, with no plausible confounders (+1)
- Very strong evidence of association-significant relative risk of >5 (<0.2) based on direct evidence with no major threats to validity (+2)
- Evidence of a dose response gradient (+1)
- All plausible confounders would have reduced the effect (+1)

Active Research

In addition to conducting a formal evidence synthesis, we conducted a survey to identify and describe current or planned research that is addressing or will address the key questions. Specific objectives were to 1) describe the data that are being collected that will help to address the key questions, 2) propose actions needed to address the key questions above within a reasonable time frame.

To identify ongoing or planned research relating to key questions, we began by sending email communications inquiring about active or planned research to groups and individuals. The groups and individuals sent initial email communications were:

- Investigators working in the areas of pain, polytrauma or TBI that were known to the Evidence Synthesis investigators or, as indicated from recent published manuscripts, are currently likely to be conducting studies in these areas. We specifically sent initial emails to several DOD researchers thought to be studying patients with polytraumatic injuries.
- Chairs of active VA workgroups, the Assessing pain in TBI workgroup (Buffum), VA Polytrauma Centers Workgroup (Clark), and the TBI QUERI Workgroup (Sayer). The PI of the current evidence synthesis project is a member of the VHA Pain Research Workgroup and sent an email communication directly to all

members of this workgroup. We also discussed this evidence synthesis project with chairs and members of these workgroups.

- Investigators of projects on polytrauma and pain identified from queries and hand-searches of several VA and non-VA website databases: (National Institutes of Health Clinical Trials data base (http:www.clinicaltrials.gov), the Computer Retrieval of Information on Scientific Projects (CRISP) database (http://crisp.cit.nih.gov/), the Meta-Register of Current Controlled Trials (http://www.controlled-trials.com/mrct/), and the VA HSR&D website (http://www.hsrd.research.va.gov/research/default.cfm).
- Each of the five HSR&D VA portfolio managers.

Email communications described our goals and the task, and asked respondents to also identify other investigators who might be working in these areas (snowball approach). Initial email messages were sent at the end of January 2008; email messages to newly identified investigators and follow-up communications occurred continuously until August 28, 2008.

PEER REVIEW

A draft version of this report was sent to the technical advisory panel and additional peer reviewers. Their comments and our responses are shown in Appendix D.

RESULTS

Literature Flow

The combined library contained 3252 citations, of which we reviewed 578 articles at the full-text level. From these, we identified systematic reviews and observational studies that addressed one or more of the key questions. Figure 2 shows the results of the literature search and the organization of themes that emerged for each key question.

Pain in Patients with Polytrauma

Figure 2. Management of Pain in Polytrauma Literature Flow

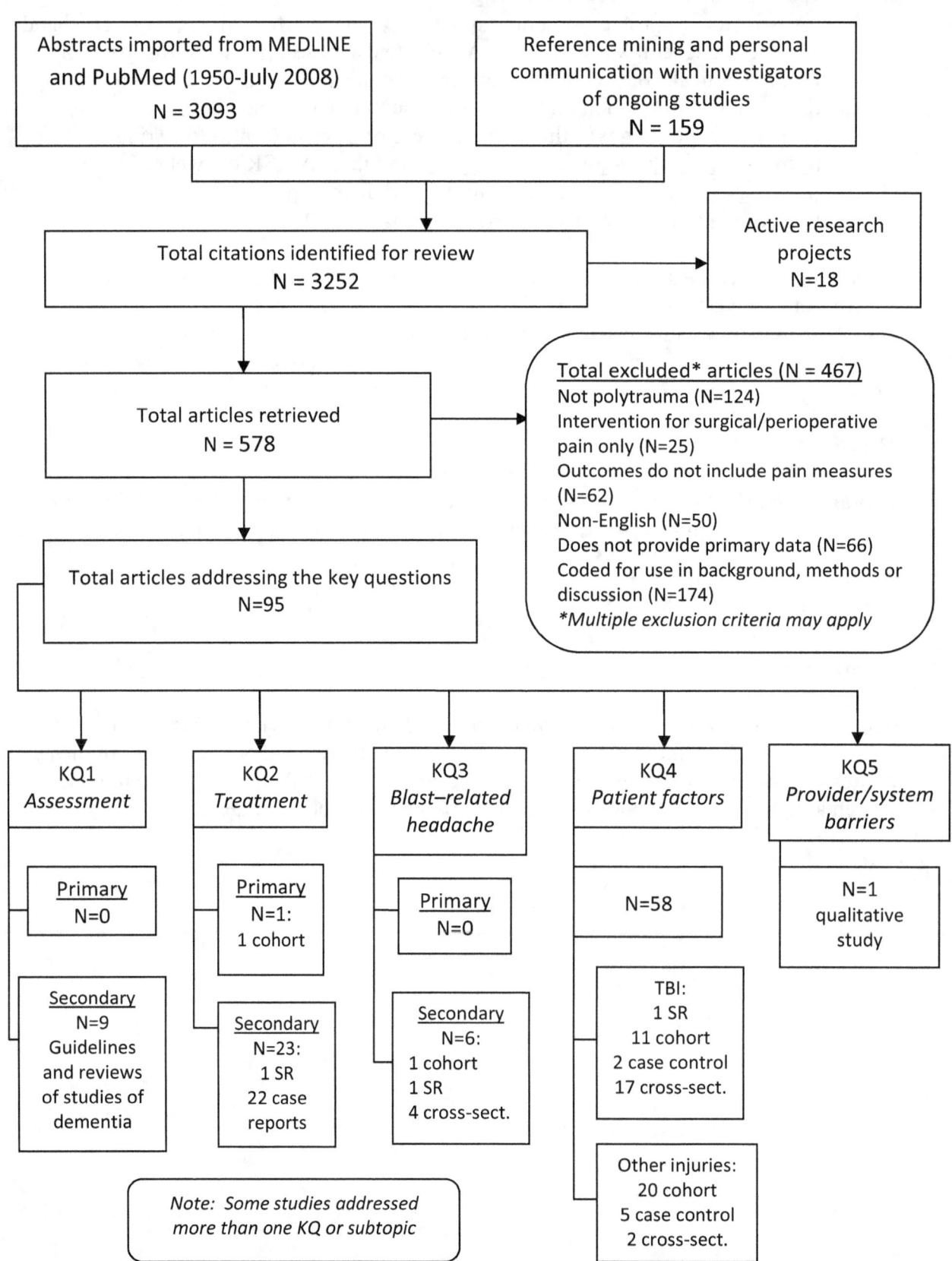

Pain in Patients with Polytrauma

Results—Key Question #1: Have reliable and valid measures and assessment tools been developed to measure pain intensity and pain-related functional interference among patients with cognitive deficits due to traumatic brain injury (TBI)? Which measures and tools are likely to be most useful in assessing pain in polytrauma patients with cognitive deficits due to TBI?

Summary of findings

There were no published studies that assessed reliability and validity of measures of pain intensity or pain-related function among patients with cognitive deficits due to TBI.

Secondary findings

- A number of primarily cross-sectional and case-control studies suggest that pain may interfere with neurocognitive functioning among TBI patients. Only some of these studies adjusted for potential confounders of the relationship between pain and neurocognitive performance.

- Several studies suggest that most individuals with cognitive impairment due to dementia can understand at least one pain self-assessment measure.

Details of Studies—Secondary Findings

Pain may interfere with neuropsychological assessment among TBI patients
We identified several narrative review articles that addressed this topic in depth.(13-15) These review articles include a number of primarily cross-sectional and case control studies that found negative associations between headache pain and cognitive functioning among TBI and non-TBI patients. Most TBI patients in these studies had mild TBI. Most of these studies support that acute or chronic pain irrespective of whether a patient has TBI, is associated with worse cognitive performance. While cognitive effects associated with pain may be quite variable, attention, memory, speed of processing and executive control may be most strongly affected.(13) Of note, investigators have identified factors other than pain that have the potential to confound or modulate the relationship between pain and neurocognitive performance. Such factors include psychological distress, mood, or anxiety disorders,(16-18) somatic complaints and concerns,(19) and sleep deprivation.(20) Thus, it remains unclear to what extent pain remains negatively associated with neurocognitive functioning when potentially confounding factors are considered.

Assessment of pain in patients with cognitive impairment due to dementia
The recently published VA Evidence Synthesis Report entitled, "Assessment and management of acute pain in adult medical inpatients: A systematic review"(21), four additional published reviews (22-25), and a guideline for assessing pain in the elderly(26) have addressed assessment of pain in patients with cognitive impairment due to dementia. Together, these reviews indicate that there is limited evidence that most individuals with mild to moderate cognitive impairment due to dementia can understand at least one self-assessment pain measure. Among the existing scales of nonverbal behavioral pain

indicators, none have been demonstrated to be substantially more reliable or valid than others for patients with cognitive impairment due to dementia. However, several of the reviews indicate that the Pain Assessment Checklist for Seniors with Limited Ability to Communicate (PACSLAC) may be especially promising or useful (27), and that the Discomfort Scale may have especially desirable psychometric properties.(28) To date, these self-assessment measures have not been specifically tested with TBI patients. Guidelines for assessing pain in patients with dementia who cannot understand any of the self-assessment measures suggest that multiple assessment methods may be best. Specific options include the use of an observational assessment measure, input from family, friends, or staff who know the patient well, and empiric pain treatment if the impaired patient has diagnoses usually associated with pain.(29-32)

Key Question #2: A. Which treatment approaches are most likely to be effective in improving pain outcomes (pain intensity and functional interference) in polytrauma patients? B. Which pain treatment approaches are most likely to enhance overall rehabilitation efforts?

Summary of findings

2A: There were no randomized controlled trials, systematic reviews, prospective cohort, case-control, or systematic observational studies that tested the efficacy or effectiveness of specific pain treatment approaches among patients with polytrauma.

2B: One fair-quality retrospective cohort study of patients who had undergone amputation at an urban trauma center demonstrated that after controlling for demographic factors, injury characteristics and other medical morbidity, inpatient rehabilitation was marginally associated with increased likelihood of return to work and decreased likelihood of reduced hours of work. (GRADE: Very Low)

Secondary Findings

- One fair-quality systematic review of primarily case reports on patients with causalgia (now known as complex regional pain syndrome II) due to war-related injuries suggests that sympathetic blocks and sympathectomy are frequently effective treatments.
- A number of manuscripts presented cases or case series describing pain treatment approaches and pain outcomes among patients with polytrauma including TBI.

Details of Studies—Primary Findings

One fair-quality retrospective cohort study of patients who underwent amputation at an urban trauma center between 1984 and 1994 examined factors that predicted whether a patient would receive inpatient rehabilitation and the success of treatment.(33) Seventy-eight patients (68% of eligible respondents) who had undergone trauma-related amputation at one hospital between 1984 and 1994 were contacted and interviewed an average of 7 years after their injuries. The study excluded amputation for non-injury reasons (e.g. diabetes), spinal cord injury or TBI. Many patients in the sample had multiple injuries. After controlling for demographic factors, injury characteristics and other medical morbidity, inpatient rehabilitation was marginally associated with increased likelihood of return to work (p=0.09) and decreased likelihood of reduced hours of work (p=0.05).

Details of Studies—Secondary Findings

One fair quality systematic review on causalgia (now known as complex regional pain syndrome II) was published in 2003.(34) In this review, MEDLINE and Index Medicus were searched using the terms, *causalgia* and *neuralgia*. All references including new cases of causalgia were included. One hundred ten manuscripts describing a total of 1,528 cases of causalgia were identified. No information about any experimental or longitudinal observational studies beyond individual cases or case series was reported. Overall, 57% of cases were war-related and 67% of cases were due to high-velocity missiles. It is unclear to what extent the overall group had polytrauma, but we infer from the traumatic nature of the injuries that polytrauma was likely common. The median nerve and sciatic trunk were the nerves most commonly involved and the most prominent clinical manifestations were burning pain (86%) diaphoresis (73%), paresthesias (96%), and sensitivity to stimuli (98%). Response to sympathetic blocks was observed in 88%, and 94% of patients undergoing sympathectomy were described as cured.

A number of manuscripts presented cases or case series describing pain treatment approaches and pain outcomes among patients with polytrauma including TBI. This information is summarized in Table 1 below. Several case reports support that intrathecal baclofen may be helpful for spasticity associated with TBI and related injuries. Despite supplemental hand-searches within our reference library for manuscripts on the use of opioids in patients with polytrauma including TBI, we found only one case report documenting (positive) specific effects of opioids in a TBI patient (included in Table 1)

Table 1—Secondary Findings pertaining to Key Question 2: Case Reports/Case Series*

Study	Study Design/ Sample	Condition(s)	Treatment Approach	Results
(35)	Single case	Severe TBI with brainstem seizures and pain	Mesothalamic electrode stimulation	Attenuated brainstem generated seizures and relieved chronic pain
(36)	Single case	TBI plus other injuries	Acupuncture	Decreased pain and anxiety
(37)	100 consecu-tive referrals	SCI (includes 15 TBI patients)	Botulinum injections and physical therapy	Clinician-reported global improvement in 90% of patients
(38)	Single case	Complex regional pain syndrome I (formerly known as Reflex sympathetic dystrophy) post-amputation	Topical capsaicin	Associated with disappearance of pain and autonomic changes
(39)	4 cases, one with TBI	Spasticity	Divalproex sodium (DVS)	Marked improvement in pain. One patient could not tolerate DVS
(40)	12 cases, 6 with missile head injury	Anxiety and headache	Fluphenazine	Reductions in headache and anxiety
(41)	2 cases, one with TBI	Central Pain	Gabapentin	*Increased* anxiety
(42)	Single case (OEF/OIF veteran)	Knee pain due to explosion, mild TBI, substance use disorder and PTSD	Multidisciplinary care including cognitive processing therapy	Decreased knee pain interference
(43)	7 cases (veterans) (5 received comparator intervention)	SCI and neuropathic pain	Healing Touch	Variable response; overall improvement in pain and satisfaction with life
(44)	Single case	Heterotopic ossification in TBI	Indomethacin and Radiation therapy	No response to indomethacin, but decreased pain with radiation therapy
(45)	Single Case	TBI with heterotopic ossification	Intense physiotherapy after surgery	Improvements in pain and behavioral symptoms
(46)	11 cases (8 with TBI)	Refractory spasticity	Intrathecal baclofen	Clinican-reported global improvement in all cases
(47)	19 patients (4 with TBI)	SCI-related spasticity	Intrathecal baclofen	Spasticity and pain improved in 14 pts.
(48)	9 cases (1 with TBI	Severe spasticity	Intrathecal baclofen	Most pts. improved, but no change in pain in TBI patient
(49)	14 cases (5 due to trauma	Spastic hypertonia	Intrathecal baclofen	Decreased pain
(50)	3 cases with TBI	Spasticity	Intrathecal baclofen	Decreased painful spasms
(51)	Single Case	TBI with unilateral central pain	Motor cortex stimulation	VAS change from 75-85 to 20-30; 50%-95% improvement in neuropathic symptoms
(52)	Single case	Severe TBI Schizophrenia	Opioid (oxycodone)	Increased interaction with others, decreased anxiety
(53)	Single case	Multiple medical conditions incl. polytrauma	Qigong Therapy	Decreased pain, weight loss, discontinuance of several medications

Study	Study Design/ Sample	Condition(s)	Treatment Approach	Results
(54)	Single case	TBI with severe headache	Sphenopalatine Ganglion pulsed radiofrequency lesioning	Long term relief of intractable headaches
(55)	10 consecutive cases (7 due to trauma)	Complex regional pain syndrome I	Spinal Cord Stimulation	Mean Numeric Rating Scale (NRS) pain score decrease of 6.2; decreased opioid use
(56)	Single case	Blast-related headache	Urea and chorionic gonadotropin	Headache free

*Subjects with TBI had moderate or severe TBI or TBI plus other injuries/complications

Key Question #3: A. Does blast-related headache pain differ in terms of phenomenology and treatment from other types of headache pain? B. Which treatments are best for persistent blast-related headache pain?

Summary of findings

There were no randomized controlled trials, cohort studies, case-control studies, or other systematic observational studies that compared patients with blast-related headache to patients with other types of headache or that specifically addressed treatments for blast-related headache pain.

Secondary findings

- Three studies (57-59) addressed the prevalence of headache among patients reporting head injuries. In a cross-sectional study of Army infantry soldiers post-deployment to Iraq with mild-TBI, most related to blast, 32% of soldiers reporting loss of consciousness and 18% of those reporting altered mental status also reported headache.(57) In a cross-sectional study of soldiers with injuries from Iraq and Afghanistan, two-thirds of whom were exposed to blast, 91% reported post-concussive symptoms, and headache was present in 47% of patients in this group.(58) Finally, in a poor-quality cohort study of civilians injured by munitions explosives in Yugoslavia, one year after injury, 30% of patients with blast injuries reported a constellation of symptoms which included headache, vertigo, and psychological and cognitive sequelae.(59)

- Two cross-sectional studies described blast injuries of the ear including hearing deficits, otalgia, and mandibular pain.(60, 61) We include this information because these types of problems have the potential to complicate the assessment and treatment of blast-related headache. In a study of service members at Walter Reed Army Medical Center referred for audiologic testing for follow-up of blast exposure, age-adjusted hearing thresholds were significantly lower than expected, 32% of patients had experienced tympanic membrane perforation, 49% reported tinnitus, and 5% reported otalgia.(60) In a study of civilians from Iran with war-related blast exposure referred to an oral/maxillofacial surgery clinic for evaluation of mandibular problems, pain was a common complaint and levels of pain were associated with distance from blasts.(61)

- We identified one good quality systematic review of post-traumatic headache in TBI,(62) but blast exposure was not included as a characteristic in any of the studies, nor did the review explore relationships between TBI severity and headache (thus we include the results here as secondary findings). The review showed that most posttraumatic headache resolves within 6-12 months, but headaches persist beyond one year in 18% to 33% of patients. Many patients with posttraumatic headache have clinical presentations similar to tension-type headache or migraine. Many clinicians treat posttraumatic headache as if they are managing primary headache.

Details of Studies—Secondary Findings

In a recent cross-sectional study assessing the prevalence and significance of self-reported history of combat-related mild TBI, soldiers from two US Army combat infantry brigades were surveyed three to four months after a yearlong deployment in Iraq in 2006.(57) Of 4,618 soldiers potentially eligible to participate, 2,714 (59%) completed surveys. The authors note that lack of availability to complete questionnaires was mostly due to normal transfers to other units, trainings or attendance at military schools. Surveys inquired whether soldiers had been injured during their deployments by a blast or explosion, a bullet, a fragment or shrapnel, a vehicle accident, or other means, and whether the injury involved the head. A soldier was considered to have mild TBI if he or she endorsed "losing consciousness," "being dazed, confused or seeing stars," or "not remembering the injury." Multivariate logistic regression analyses were used to identify correlates of a range of self-reported outcomes including general health, missed workdays, medical visits, and somatic and postconcussive symptoms. Of soldiers reporting injuries with loss of consciousness or altered mental status, 75% reported being exposed to blast or explosion. Five percent reported injury with loss of consciousness, 10% reported in juries with altered mental status, and 17% reported other injuries during deployment. Headache was common, present in 32% of those reporting injury with loss of consciousness and 18% of those reporting altered mental status, as compared to soldiers who reported other injuries (12%) or no injury (8%) (p<0.001). In models adjusted for demographics, mechanism of injury, blast exposure, post-traumatic stress disorder (PTSD), depression, combat intensity, and hospitalization, the odds of headache remained significantly greater in soldiers reporting loss of consciousness versus other injury: 2.38 (1.12-5.07). The odds of headache were not significantly greater in soldiers reporting altered mental status vs. other injury: 1.63 (0.92-2.90). Overall, the analyses show that, except for in the case of headache when there is loss of consciousness, the associations among TBI and physical health problems are no longer significant when PTSD and depression are included in models.

An abstract from a cross-sectional study described the characteristics of soldiers returning from Iraq or Afghanistan who were injured in a blast, fall, gun shot wound, or motor vehicle accident, and screened for TBI by the Defense and Veterans Brain Injury Center (DVBIC) of Walter Reed Army Medicine Center between January 2003 and April

Pain in Patients with Polytrauma

2005.(58) The sample included the initial 433 patients seen by the DVIBC. The sample was 95% males, modal age 21. Sixty-eight percent reported blast exposure, 79% reported loss of consciousness less than one hour, and 43% reported post-traumatic amnesia less than 24 hours. Ninety-one percent of patients reported post-concussive symptoms. Headache (47%), memory deficits (46%), and irritability/aggression (41%) were the most common post-concussive symptoms.

A poor-quality cohort study of 1,303 civilians who had been injured by munitions explosives in Yugoslavia between 1991 and 1994 and admitted to the US Military Medical Academy in Belgrade assessed the effects of blast exposure within one year of injury.(59) Approximately 30% of patients with 665 blast injuries reported persisting symptoms including headache, vertigo, positive Romberg's sign, retrograde amnesia, mental blockage, apathy/lethargy, psychomotor agitation, and anxiety. The study was limited by inadequate reporting on rates of follow-up, timing of follow-up assessment, or details of the measurement of these symptoms.

An observational study that sought to examine whether blast was related to significant hearing changes collected audiologic data on 258 service members.(60) The investigators also explored whether polytraumatic injuries were associated with hearing loss. Potential subjects were referred for audiologic testing at Walter Reed Army Medical Center as part of a standard protocol for soldiers reporting at least one blast-related exposure. Only 162 out of 258 patients (63%) had hearing test data available for review. The mean age was 29 years and 98% were male. Within this group, age-adjusted actual hearing thresholds were significantly lower than expected, and 32% of patients had experienced tympanic membrane perforation, 49% reported tinnitus, and 5% reported otalgia. There was no association between polytrauma status and other characteristics. A cross-sectional study of 495 civilians with blast exposure who were referred to an oral/maxillofacial surgery clinic from the Medical Services Centre for War Injured Patients in Tehran, Iran between March 1984 and February 1990 reported that pain was a common complaint and that levels of pain were associated with distance from blasts.(61) In 115 patients, pain was localized in the external acoustic meatus and 15 patients complained of total facial pain. Forty-nine percent of the sample "responded" to limiting jaw movement, adopting a soft-diet, and the use of "pain killers," and 77% responded to a combination of "pain killers" and muscle relaxants. Patient characteristics and the timing and methods to measure outcomes were not specified.

Finally, we identified one good quality systematic review of post-traumatic headache in TBI.(62) In this review, the investigators searched MEDLINE for literature on posttraumatic headache published between January 1990 and February 2005. Five studies specifically describing patient characteristics and types of headache were identified.(63-67) The total number of subjects in these studies was 423 patients. Blast exposure was not included as a characteristic in any of the five studies, and the review did not explore relationships between TBI severity and headache. The review showed that posttraumatic headache usually resolves within 6-12 months, but that 18% to 33% of the time, headaches persist beyond one year. Many (37%) of patients with posttraumatic headache had clinical presentations similar to tension-type headache or migraine (29%). Many clinicians treat posttraumatic headache as if they were managing primary headache. The authors conclude that there is no universally accepted protocol for treating posttraumatic headache, and that randomized controlled trials are needed in this area.

Key Question #4. What patient factors are associated with better and worse (pain-related) clinical outcomes among polytrauma patients? Have interventions been developed to specifically address these factors?

Summary of Findings

There were no randomized controlled trials. One systematic review, 11 cohort, 2 case-control, and 17 cross-sectional studies specifically addressed patient factors associated with outcomes in TBI patients. Twenty cohort, 2 cross-sectional, and 5 case-control studies addressed patient factors associated with outcomes in other polytrauma patients. Evidence Table 1 in Appendix E shows the data abstracted from these studies.

Traumatic Brain Injury
- One recent fair-quality systematic review showed that overall, 58% of patients with TBI have chronic headache, and that brain injury is associated with headache even after adjustment for post-traumatic stress disorder (PTSD).(68) These findings are consistent with our review, which included additional manuscripts, which found that among patients with TBI, headache is present in one-third to one-half of patients up to five years after injury. (GRADE: Low)

- The recent fair-quality systematic review above also found that patients with mild TBI were more likely to have headache than patients with moderate or severe TBI.(68) However, our review showed very mixed findings regarding the association between severity of TBI and pain (GRADE: Very Low).

- Psychological factors, including depression and posttraumatic stress disorder (PTSD), insomnia and fatigue are associated with pain in TBI patients. (GRADE: Low)

Other injuries in polytrauma patients
- Characteristics of injuries (location, severity, and whether they are multiple) are associated with clinical outcomes including persistent pain and functional status. Specific factors associated with worse pain-related outcomes include: multiple injuries, foot injuries or injuries below the knee joint, and concurrent head injury or cognitive disability. (GRADE: Low)

- Other factors associated with better outcomes in some studies of patients with polytraumatic injuries other than TBI were younger age, higher educational achievement, having a white collar job or higher income. (GRADE: Very Low)

Pain in Patients with Polytrauma

Details of Studies—Traumatic Brain Injury

Prevalence of pain and headache among TBI patients
One fair-quality systematic review was published in 2008. In this review, Ovid/MEDLINE, PubMed, and MD consult databases were searched using the terms *brain injury, pain, headache, blast injury, combat, combat disorders, war, military medicine, wounds and injuries, military personnel,* and *veterans*. The Cochrane Collaboration, National Institutes of Health Clinical Trials Database, Meta-register of Current Controlled Trials and CRISP database were searched using the term *brain injury*. Articles were included which were published between 1951 and February 2008 (however one article from 1939 is also included in the review.(69) The search was not limited by language or publication status. Case reports and review articles were cited only if no other data were available. Twenty-three studies (15 cross-sectional, 5 prospective observational, and 3 retrospective observational) including 4,206 patients were identified. No randomized clinical trials were identified. Data were pooled across studies to obtain overall prevalence rates. The review showed that 58% (95%CI 55.5-60.2%) of patients with TBI have chronic headache, and that brain injury is associated with headache even after adjustment for post-traumatic stress disorder (PTSD).(68)

In our review, we found seven prospective and one retrospective cohort studies that report on the prevalence of pain and headache among TBI patients.(70-77) In a good-quality prospective cohort study of 146 patients enrolled in acute inpatient rehabilitation for TBI, 73% reported pain at one year and 55% reported interference from pain.(71) One fair-quality prospective cohort study measured prevalence and type of headache among 109 patients with moderate to severe TBI consecutively admitted to one of four VA Polytrauma Rehabilitation Centers (PRCs) over 12 months.(70) On admission, 38% of patients reported headache. Sixty-four percent of patients with headache reported no to mild levels of incapacitation from headaches. Among patients with headaches at admission, 54% reported persistent headache symptoms at six months, and of this group, 96% still had headaches at 12 months. Of patients without headache at admission, the majority remained headache free over 12 months. In a fair-quality prospective cohort study of 161 patients admitted to a brain injury rehabilitation unit, 62% reported some type of pain and 31% reported daily pain or continuous pain at six months.(72) Headache was the most frequently reported type of pain. In a fair-quality prospective cohort study of 231 patients admitted to three trauma centers in France with severe head injuries reassessed five years after injury, the prevalence of headache was 44 to 54%, significantly greater than 16% in a comparison group with lower limb injury but no TBI.(73) In a poor quality prospective cohort study of patients with TBI consecutively admitted to an inpatient urban rehabilitation program who completed follow-up assessments, headache prevalence increased from 31% 2 years post-injury to 42% 5 years post-injury.(76) In a poor-quality prospective cohort study of 132 patients consecutively admitted to an inpatient TBI rehabilitation center, 10% of patients had co-existing peripheral nerve injuries, and of these patients, 31% reported pain.(77) In a poor-quality retrospective cohort study of 200 patients admitted to an inpatient accident service, headaches persisted in 17 to 18% of cases 6 months after injury.(75) Finally, in another poor-quality retrospective cohort

Pain in Patients with Polytrauma

study, 58% of patients admitted to an Australian teaching hospital had headaches 5 years after TBI.(74)

Two fair-quality case-control studies demonstrated that pain is more common or more severe in TBI patients than other populations.(78, 79) One of these studies showed that overall pain scores were higher in a volunteer community sample of mild to severe TBI patients at least 12-months post-injury compared to a group of non-injured controls (17.2 vs. 10.1, on a scale of 0-78 using the McGill pain questionnaire,p=.013).(78) The other study showed that the prevalence of pain complaints was 59% in a sample of patients with TBI referred for neuropsychological assessment at a medical center versus 22% of non-TBI patients also referred for neuropsychological assessment (p<.001).(79)

Several cross-sectional studies also support that pain and headache are common among TBI patients.(57, 58, 80-86) In these studies, pain was present in 22% to 90% of patients. In one of these studies of young patients admitted to a brain injury rehabilitation ward in London an average of 25 weeks after injury, only 12% reported headache.(82) Headache was the most common type of pain complaint according to two of these studies.(81, 85) Another study found that reflex sympathetic dystrophy (now known as Complex Regional Pain Syndrome I) was present in 13 of 100 patients consecutively admitted to an inpatient brain injury unit.(84) Notably, in several(81, 85, 86) of the above studies, case status was established at the time of outpatient follow-up assessment; thus, patients with persisting pain complaints may be overrepresented in these samples.

Taken together these studies show that pain is common among patients with TBI, present in approximately one-third to one-half of patients up to five years after injury. One prospective cohort, and several cross-sectional studies suggest that headache is the most common pain complaint among TBI patients.

Relationship between severity of TBI and pain in TBI patients
One fair-quality systematic review was published in 2008. In this review, Ovid/MEDLINE, PubMed, and MD consult databases were searched using the terms *brain injury, pain, headache, blast injury, combat, combat disorders, war, military medicine, wounds and injuries, military personnel,* and *veterans*. The Cochrane Collaboration, National Institutes of Health Clinical Trials Database, Meta-register of Current Controlled Trials and CRISP database were searched using the term *brain injury*. Articles were included which were published between 1951 and February 2008 (however one article from 1939 is also included in the review.(69) The search was not limited by language or publication status. Case reports and review articles were cited only if no other data were available. Twenty-three studies (15 cross-sectional, 5 prospective observational, and 3 retrospective observational) including 4,206 patients were identified. No randomized clinical trials were identified. Data were pooled across studies to obtain overall prevalence rates. The review showed that among civilians, the prevalence of chronic pain was 51.5% (95%CI 49.8% - 53.2%) among patients with mild TBI, compared with 32.1% (95%CI 29.3% - 34.9%) among patients with moderate or severe TBI.(68)

Pain in Patients with Polytrauma

In our review, which included a number of studies not included in the systematic review above, one fair-quality prospective cohort study of 109 patients admitted to one of four VA PRCs, no statistically significant relationships were identified between Glasgow Coma Scale (GCS) score, Loss of Consciousness (LOC), or duration of post-traumatic amnesia (all indicators of head injury severity) and posttraumatic headache prevalence.(70) One good-quality prospective cohort study of 146 patients enrolled in a University acute inpatient rehabilitation program similarly found that baseline GCS was not associated with pain status one year after injury.(71) In another fair-quality prospective cohort study of 231 patients admitted to French trauma centers with severe head injuries who were reassessed five years after injury, headache prevalence was not found to be significantly different according to head injury severity.(73) Patients with severe head injury were less likely to complete follow-up assessments due to deaths. In an additional prospective cohort study of 200 consecutive individuals admitted to an urban hospital with head injuries, headache persisting longer than two months was not more prevalent among patients with more severe head injuries than patients with milder head injuries.(87) Finally, a poor-quality retrospective cohort study of 200 patients admitted to an inpatient accident service found no differences in the prevalence of headache when comparing patients with mild head injury to those with moderate to severe TBI three and six months after injury.(75)

In a cross-sectional study of consecutive TBI patients seen in an outpatient brain injury clinic, over half of the sample reported chronic pain (primarily headaches), and there were similar rates of pain reports when comparing patients with mild TBI to patients with more severe TBI.(81) A retrospective review of the records of 200 consecutive cases of head injury admitted to the surgical wards of the Edinburgh Royal Infirmary similarly found no increase in headache prevalence among patients who had presented with milder head injuries.(88) Finally, in a cross-sectional examination of the validity of the SF-36 for characterizing outcome after multiple trauma, there were no differences in the SF-36 bodily pain scale based on severity of head trauma among patients discharged from trauma centers who did not have concurrent orthopedic injuries.(89)

However, one fair-quality retrospective cohort study,(90) one fair-quality case-control study (79) and five studies using cross-sectional designs(82, 85, 86, 91, 92) found a higher prevalence of headache among patients with mild TBI as compared to more severe TBI. In the retrospective cohort study of 228 patients a median of four years after being admitted to a university ICU for major trauma, patients with severe head injury were less likely to report problems with pain/discomfort (OR 0.31, 95%CI 0.15 - 0.64) after adjusting for retrospectively-patient-reported baseline levels of symptoms and functioning. However, patients with severe head injury were less likely to participate in the follow-up surveys. In five of case-control and cross-sectional studies, study samples were established from referrals or attendees of outpatient follow-up clinics for TBI. Generally, patients were seen in these follow up clinics between six months and two years after their injuries. In one of the studies, the sample consisted of patients admitted to a subacute rehabilitation unit on average 25 weeks post-injury,(82) and in the remaining study, it was unclear whether the study cohort was established at the time of injury or time of outpatient follow-up.(92) Overall, this group of studies found that patients with mild TBI who attend outpatient brain injury clinics are two to three times more likely to report headache than patients with moderate or severe TBI. However, the analyses in these studies were not adjusted for potential confounding factors, and specific reasons why patients were referred to or sought care in these settings were not specified or adjusted for in most of the studies.

In summary, there is very limited evidence showing that patients with mild TBI are more likely to have headache or other pain than patients without TBI. While one retrospective cohort, one case-control, and a number of cross-sectional studies suggest that patients with mild TBI may be more likely to have headache pain than patients with moderate or severe TBI, six prospective cohort studies and additional cross-sectional studies did not find such a relationship. In the single systematic review showing a difference in rates of pain across levels of TBI severity, data were pooled across studies using different patient samples and designs. Most of the studies identified in that review and in our review that found associations between milder head injury and headache were done in outpatient settings, up to several years post-injury, and did not adjust for potential confounders that may influence relationships between TBI severity and pain. On the other hand, most of the samples in the identified cohort studies were assembled at the time of admission to a hospital or inpatient rehabilitation setting. It is therefore likely that differences in sample composition contribute to the differences in findings between the cross-sectional and cohort studies; patients with mild TBI may be more likely to be referred to or attend outpatient follow-up appointments when they have bothersome or persistent symptoms such as headache.

<u>Relationships between other patient factors and pain outcomes in patients with TBI</u>
Demographics: There are mixed findings regarding the association between demographic factors and pain outcomes in TBI patients. In one good-quality prospective cohort study of 146 patients enrolled in a university acute inpatient rehabilitation program, pain one year after injury was significantly associated with being female and non-white; being non-white remained significantly associated with reports of pain at one year in a multivariate regression model (taking other factors into account).(71) However, a fair-quality cohort study of veterans at VA PRCs(70) and a cross-sectional study of outpatients referred for neuropsychological evaluation (93) did not detect significant associations between demographic factors and headache frequency.

Blast exposure: In a cross-sectional study of 188 service members admitted to one of four VA PRCs, blast exposure was not found to be a significant predictor of pain.(80)

Psychological factors: In a fair-quality prospective cohort study of 109 patients admitted to one of four VA PRCs, headache density (a measure combining headache-related incapacitation and frequency) at six and 12 months was associated with higher depression and anxiety levels among patients with persistent headaches, and among patients with delayed onset headaches.(70) In another good-quality prospective cohort study of 146 patients enrolled in a university acute inpatient rehabilitation program, depression one year after injury remained significantly associated with reports of pain at one year (taking other factors into account).(71) Depression was also found to be a significant factor mediating the relationship between pain and community participation. In a fair-quality prospective cohort study of 161 patients admitted to a tertiary care center brain injury rehabilitation unit, frequency but not severity of chronic pain was associated with PTSD (p<.05).(72) In a multivariate model including psychological factors, only avoidant coping style remained significantly associated with pain severity after controlling for PTSD severity. In a fair-quality prospective cohort study of 47 patients admitted to a regional trauma center, pain was found to be highly correlated with depression (r=.81) in post hoc analyses. Finally, in a cross-sectional study of 84 patients from eight outpatient Mid-west rehabilitation centers, in a model including perceived stress, impact of events, and litigation status, pain was significantly associated with depression (partial R^2 = .07, p=.001).(94)

Fatigue and Insomnia: In a poor-quality prospective cohort study of 38 TBI patients admitted to an inpatient rehabilitation service, there were highly significant correlations between levels of fatigue and pain at one and 2 years post-injury (R=.49 and .62, respectively, p<.01).(95) Another fair-quality case-control study of community volunteers showed that fatigue was correlated with the SF-36 bodily pain scale in TBI patients (R=.389, p<.011).(78) In another fair-quality case-control study of patients referred to a university outpatient neuropsychology service, pain was highly associated with insomnia (p<.001).(79) In an additional cross-sectional study of Canadian community volunteers, pain frequency was significantly associated with insomnia in TBI patients; pain remained a significant predictor of insomnia in a multivariate model that included depression, severity of injury and fatigue.(96) Finally, in another cross-sectional study, pain was significantly associated with insomnia in TBI patients admitted to a comprehensive outpatient rehabilitation program; however, pain dropped out of a multivariate model in which presence of insomnia was the outcome.(97)

Taken together, this group of studies provides limited evidence that psychological factors, including depression and posttraumatic stress disorder (PTSD), insomnia and fatigue are associated with pain in TBI patients.

Details of Studies —Other Injuries in Polytrauma Patients

Injury characteristics—amputations: Studies support that injury factors (location, severity, multiplicity) are often associated with pain-related outcomes in patients with amputations. In a fair-quality retrospective cohort study of 78 trauma-related amputation patients, many of whom had multiple trauma, greater initial severity of injury was associated with significantly worse self-reported physical functioning including bodily pain.(33) In another fair-quality retrospective cohort study, investigators studied 326 patients from Belgrade who experienced missile-caused peripheral nerve lesions, some of whom likely had multiple trauma.(98, 99) In multivariate analyses, three factors were significant predictors of pain up to five years after injury: type of pain syndrome (e.g., complex regional pain syndrome II or deafferentation pain), severity of initial nerve injury, and an absence of pain paroxysms. In an additional fair-quality retrospective cohort study examining the long-term results of compartment syndrome, polytrauma patients were compared to those with a single injury.(100) The investigators did not find a difference with respect to strength, pain, or function and concluded that secondary injuries did not negatively impact the outcome of compartment syndrome. A poor-quality retrospective cohort study compared functional outcomes of Vietnam Veterans who had isolated transtibial amputations to those with amputations and at least one other major injury.(101) The polytrauma group scored significantly lower than the control group on all 8 subscale scores of the SF-36 including bodily pain, whereas quality of life scores from the single trauma group did not differ with those from the control group. A poor-quality quality case-control study compared 23 bilateral Vietnam Veteran amputees to age and gender matched controls from a national registry. Cases were surveyed an average of 28 years after injury. This study showed that while overall physical function was lower in the case group, bodily pain scores were not significantly different.(102) Finally, a cross-sectional study provided descriptive data on stump pain, phantom sensation, and phantom pain in 40 civilians from Sierra Leone who suffered traumatic upper limb amputation in a civil war setting.(103) Interviews were conducted 10-48 months post-injury. All amputees (100%) had stump pain in the last month and 93% had phantom sensations. Phantom pain was less common among patients with bilateral than unilateral amputations (18% versus 38%; no p-value reported). In an additional cross-sectional study of civilian amputees, stump and phantom limb pain were reported by 73% of multiple level amputees as compared to 63% of upper limb and 74% of lower limb amputees (no comparison significance tests reported).(104)

Injury characteristics—orthopedic injuries Studies also suggest that injury factors are associated with pain-related outcomes in patients with orthopedic injuries. A good-quality retrospective cohort study of 389 patients compared long-term functional outcomes among 3 groups, based on the site of fracture: above-knee, below knee, or combined fractures above and below the knee.(105) A mean of 17 years after injury (minimum 10 years), although persistent pain was not significantly more frequent among patients with below-knee fractures compared with above-knee fractures (46% v. 39%, p=0.25), persistent pain was significantly more common in patients with combined injuries as compared to fractures about the knee joint (58.5% vs. 39.3%, p<.001). Two additional small, fair-quality case-control studies compared functional outcomes in small numbers of polytrauma patients with and without foot injuries.(106, 107) In both studies, the outcomes of multiply injured patients with foot injuries were significantly worse than that of patients without foot injuries. Patients with foot injuries had a dramatically lower scores on SF-36 scales of physical function, role physical (perception of physical functioning), bodily pain, and social function compared to controls.(106, 107)

In another fair-quality prospective cohort study, 659 patients with multiple orthopedic injuries were compared to 165 patients with orthopedic injuries plus other types of injuries.(108) Six months post-injury, patients with combined orthopedic and other injuries had greater pain intensity and reported more disability than patients with multiple orthopedic injuries alone. A fair-quality retrospective cohort study compared pain and function in 27 long-term survivors of open pelvic fracture with the experience of 84 survivors of closed pelvic fracture.(109) Subjects were multiple system blunt trauma patients with a pelvic fracture, and associated injuries included head injury, thoracic trauma, abdominal injury, extremity fractures, and spinal fractures. Survivors of open pelvic fracture had non-significantly lower SF-36 bodily pain scores, and significantly lower scores for physical functioning and role physical subscales, indicating worse outcomes. Finally, a fair-quality prospective cohort study of orthopedic injuries was conducted in 830 polytrauma patients with spine injury.(110) Degree of injury severity was correlated with pain, functional independence, and return to employment one year and two years follow-up.

Injury characteristics—other polytraumatic injuries: A number of additional cohort studies examined relationships between various injury characteristics and functional outcomes including or in addition to measures of pain.(109, 111-120) Pain intensity was not a main outcome in these studies and was often measured using a subscale of a functional status measure. In only some of these studies were potentially confounding factors adjusted for in analyses involving pain outcomes.(113-115, 119) Most of the studies did not have excessive loss to follow-up, and some studies determined that patients lost to follow-up were not substantially different from patients represented in the study.(112, 113, 115, 116, 120) Almost all of the studies that compared multiply and singly injured patients to patients with a single injury, or measured the severity of injury, found an association between multiple or severe single injuries and worse functional outcomes and pain.(111, 112, 114-118) Some studies that included patients with cognitive disabilities or head injuries found associations between head injury or cognitive disability and decreased functional outcome.(112-115, 117) In an additional poor-quality case control study of 49 patients (setting not specified), patients with head injury plus other types of polytrauma were not found to have worse bodily pain at 6 or 12 months after injury compared to patients with TBI alone.(121) Finally, other injury characteristics associated with worse functional and pain outcomes were lower limb injuries,(114, 116, 120)longer hospital length of stay,(115) and admission to intensive care unit (ICU) and length of ICU stay.

In summary, many cohort studies as well as several case-control and cross-sectional studies found that polytraumatic injury characteristics (principally location, initial severity, and multiplicity of injury) are associated with pain and functional outcomes over time. Injuries below the knee joint are associated with worse outcomes compared to injuries above the knee in polytrauma patients. A number of these studies did not adjust for factors that may confound relationships between injury characteristics and pain-related outcomes.

Demographics: A number of manuscripts reported adjusting for demographic variables (mainly age) in multivariate analyses, but did not report whether and to what extent these variables were significantly associated with pain outcomes. One good-quality (115) and three fair-quality (33, 112, 118) cohort studies found associations between younger age and better functional outcomes in polytrauma patients. One good-quality cohort study (115) and one fair-quality cohort study (111) found associations between being male and better functional outcomes. In an additional cross-sectional study of 40 civilians from Sierra Leone who suffered traumatic upper limb amputation, phantom pain was more common in women than men (63% versus 25%, p=0.057).(103) However, in one fair-quality prospective cohort study of 62 patients injured in traffic accidents, there were no significant differences in SF-36 bodily pain scores by gender in bivariate analyses two and eight months post-injury.(122) Finally, in one fair-quality retrospective cohort study of 78 trauma-related amputation patients, being white was associated with better SF-36 PCS and bodily pain outcome scores, higher likelihood of return to work, and lower likelihood of reduced work hours.(33)

Other factors associated with better functional status were higher educational achievement (two good-quality (115, 119) and one fair quality (114) cohort studies), having a professional/white collar job (one good quality (119) and two fair-quality (112, 118) cohort studies) and higher income, job stability, job flexibility and lower physical demands at work (one good quality cohort study).(119) The authors of this latter study also found an association between receiving worker's compensation and lower return to work rate.

Psychosocial Factors: Almost no studies reported on the relationships between psychosocial factors and pain-related outcomes in patients with polytraumatic injuries other than TBI. In one fair-quality retrospective cohort study of 69 patients admitted to an inpatient surgical service, loss of non-work activities was significantly correlated with pain.(112) One cross-sectional study provided descriptive data on stump pain, phantom sensation, and phantom pain 10-48 months post-injury in 40 civilians from Sierra Leone who had suffered traumatic upper limb amputation in a civil war setting.(103) No significant relationships were reported between mood and the prevalence of phantom or stump pain.

To summarize, there is very limited evidence regarding the extent to which demographic factors are associated with pain-related outcomes in patients with polytraumatic injuries other than TBI. Four cohort studies show that younger age is associated with better longer-term outcomes in patients with severe multiple injuries, and three cohort studies and one cross-sectional study show a relationship between male sex and improved outcomes after major trauma. There is almost no information available regarding relationships between race and ethnicity and pain-related outcomes. There is almost no information available regarding relationships between psychosocial factors and pain-related outcomes in patients with polytraumatic injuries other than TBI.

Key Question #5. What are unique provider and system barriers to detecting and treating pain among polytrauma patients? Have interventions been developed to effectively address these barriers?

Summary of findings

There were no randomized controlled trials, cohort studies, case-control studies, or other systematic observational studies that addressed provider and system barriers to detecting and treating pain among polytrauma patients. One qualitative study of providers from four VA Polytrauma Rehabilitation Centers (PRCs) addressed potential provider and system barriers to treating polytrauma patients.(3) In qualitative interviews, providers reported that polytrauma patients are very complex to treat, and that the work with this population is very challenging and emotionally taxing. Increasing use of multidisciplinary and concurrent care, and consultation from experts may be necessary to provide the complex care that is needed.

Details of Study

Pain in Patients with Polytrauma

This study was a qualitative study of provider perspectives on the rehabilitation of patients with polytrauma. This study which used Rapid Assessment Process methodology including semi-structured interviews, observation, and field liaison. The purpose of the study was to describe, from the perspective of providers working or affiliated with one of four VA Polytrauma Rehabilitation Centers (PRCs), 1) patients with combat-related polytrauma and their rehabilitation; 2) polytrauma patient family member involvement in rehabilitation; and 3) the impact on providers of providing polytrauma rehabilitation. Clinicians of various disciplines were selected among the four PRC sites, as well as personnel who work closely with the PRCs, including: 1) clinicians who provide regular consultation to PRC patients, including pain, PTSD, infectious disease, and low-vision specialists; 2) military liaisons who are US Department of Defense (DOD) employees housed at the PRC to help active-duty patients navigate across care systems; and 3) the VA points of contact who help US Service members obtain needed VA services; specific demographics of the clinicians interviewed were not provided. Fifty-six interviews were conducted.

A number of common themes were identified which are pertinent to this key question:
1. Patients with blast-related injuries including TBI have more injuries and more severe injuries than other patient populations. Serious psychiatric disorders, including PTSD and injury-related pain are highly prevalent, and complicate rehabilitation for TBI. These factors make this patient population quite complex to treat.
2. Providers find working with this population very challenging and emotionally taxing.
3. In order to address the level of complexity, providers are increasingly using co-treatment across disciplines, more regular consultation with services outside rehabilitation, such as surgery, amputation care, and psychiatry, and more frequent consultation with colleagues within and across the PRCs. PRC teams are expanding to include experts in areas including pain.
4. Spouses, parents, siblings, and children have become intensely involved in the injured service member's rehabilitation and have their own informational, instrumental, and support needs. Providers must respond to family needs and engage them as collaborators in the rehabilitation process.

Limitations—Literature Review

Heterogeneity and Generalizability

Due to innumerable etiologies and combinations of injuries, there is great heterogeneity among polytrauma patients. For example, within the category of blast-related head injury alone, there are multiple potential mechanisms of brain injury, and injuries may or may not be concurrent with other penetrating head injuries.(123) There is consequent heterogeneity among the study samples described in the literature as well as in the methods used to describe study samples. Many studies were done at single sites or within specialized types of settings. Thus, the conclusions we might draw from a particular study or set of studies may have limited relevance for other polytrauma patients, and comparisons among studies may be challenging.

Scope

Due in part to the degree of heterogeneity among studies and their descriptions, as well as the lack of precision inherent in the term, "polytrauma", we adopted a fairly stringent operational definition for polytrauma (multiple concurrent injuries in two or more systems) and focused on identifying studies that clearly included majorities of patients with polytrauma in their samples. Thus, for example, some studies of patients with spinal cord injuries or amputations were not included unless there was clear indication at the abstract or full-text level that multiple injuries were (often) involved. It is therefore likely that some manuscripts that might have relevance for the treatment of pain in polytrauma or subgroups of polytrauma patients were not identified. Surgical approaches were excluded due to the heterogeneity of the conditions being treated with specific techniques. We did not feel that information generated from review of specific surgical approaches would be very generalizable to the polytrauma patient population as a whole. We note that we did search more broadly for studies pertaining to TBI and blast since there is particular relevance for a large segment of the OEF/OIF patient population.

Publication Bias

Our search strategies were comprehensive and we evaluated a large number of studies for possible inclusion in the review. Two librarians independently searched the literature and their results were combined to form our reference library. While this process identified many manuscripts for potential inclusion in the review, it is possible that our search terms did not capture some relevant manuscripts, especially for older studies which might not have been indexed in databases as pertaining to polytrauma or multiple injury/trauma. We therefore included additional search terms pertaining to blast, TBI, and war, and relied extensively on reference lists of studies, review articles, editorials, and consulting experts to identify additional manuscripts for review.

Study quality

We did not exclude individual studies based on quality rating alone. Thus the strength of our conclusions is inherently limited by the quality variation among included studies. We did make an effort to note particular methodologic limitations, and each cohort and case-control study was closely reviewed for overall quality using a rigorously developed approach. Although cross-sectional studies were not formally rated, methodologic limitations were often noted.

RESULTS—ACTIVE RESEARCH

Summary of findings

Nineteen relevant active or planned projects were identified and project data were collected on 18 of these projects. Pain measures constitute main outcomes in 8 of the studies, and will be collected as secondary outcomes in 10 of the studies. Fifteen of the studies should generate information regarding patient factors that may contribute to pain-related outcomes among polytrauma patients (Key Question 4), and 4 studies are testing interventions for pain among polytrauma patients (Key Question 2). One study will test the reliability and validity of measures to assess pain in cognitively-impaired TBI patients and another study is using primarily qualitative methods to examine the utility of a CPRS pain assessment template module to assist clinicians in evaluating pain in PRC patients with cognitive impairment (Key Question 1). One study is examining the phenomenology and treatment of blast vs. other types of headache (Key Question 3), and one study is addressing provider and systems barriers to detecting and treating pain in polytrauma patients (Key Question 5).

Details of findings

Email communications were sent to a total of 73 individuals, 4 VA workgroups (via their chairs), and 5 HSR&D portfolio managers, inquiring about possible projects the addressing key questions and inquiring about identifying others who might be doing or planning research relevant to the key questions. Individual email recipients included 41 VA investigators, 5 Department of Defense (DOD) investigators, and 27 non-VA, non-DOD investigators. Responses were received from 47 investigators. Nineteen relevant projects were identified and project data were collected on 18 of these projects. Table 2 on the following pages lists the ongoing studies for which data were available. The characteristics of these studies are described in further detail in Appendix E, Evidence Table 2.

Pain in Patients with Polytrauma

Table 2. Summary of active research studies of pain in polytrauma

Title of Project	Main objective(s) of project	Pain-related variable(s) main or secondary outcome?	Study characteristics	KQ
Concurrent Validity of 4 Pain Intensity Scales in persons with Polytrauma and Cognitive Impairment(124)	Examine the concurrent validity of four pain intensity scales in the traumatic brain injury (TBI) inpatient rehabilitation population	Main	Study design: prospective randomized measurement study Sample: 15 TBI patients	1
Pain Assessment in Polytrauma Rehabilitation Centers (PRCs)(125)	Evaluate utility of CPRS pain assessment templates, modify education materials; develop pain reports for clinicians and pain assessment database; identify best practices for pain care	Main	Study design: Qualitative Sample: Providers and nursing staff in two PRCs	1,5
Evaluation of Stepped Care for Chronic Pain (ESCAPE)(126)	Compare a stepped care intervention vs. usual care in OIF/OEF veterans with chronic and disabling musculoskeletal pain	Main	Study design: RCT Sample: 300 OIF/OEF veterans	2,4
The ViRTICo Trial: Virtual Reality Therapy & Imaging in Combat Veterans(127)	Compare effects of Virtual Reality Exposure Therapy & Imaging compared with Prolonged Exposure (current first-line therapy)	Secondary	Study design: controlled clinical trial Sample: OEF/OIF veterans with PTSD and TBI combined; PTSD alone; TBI alone; neither PTSD or TBI.	2,4
Regional Anesthesia Military Battlefield Pain Outcomes Study(128)	Determine short-term and long-term pain-related outcomes in OEF/OIF veterans with traumatic extremity injuries; evaluate efficacy of early aggressive advanced regional anesthetic interventional techniques 2-yrs post-injury	Main	Study design: prospective cohort Sample: OEF/OIF soldiers with one or more maligned or amputated limbs	2,4
Chronic Headache among OEF/OIF Veterans Exposed to Blasts(129)	Evaluate initial characteristics and treatment of blast-TBI in OEF/OIF veterans; assess feasibility and effectiveness of brief cognitive-behavioral headache management treatment (BCBHMT)	Main	Study design: case series Sample: OEF/OIF veterans	2,3
Headaches in veterans returning from Iraq/Afghanistan: relation to trauma and combat-related injury(130)	To determine the relationship between Post-Traumatic Stress Disorder (PTSD), TBI, self-report of headaches, and combat-related injury in Operation Enduring Freedom (OEF) and Operation Iraqi Freedom (OIF) veterans	Main	Study design: Cross-sectional Sample: 343 male and female veterans registering for care	4
Long-term Outcomes in Burned OEF/OIF Veterans (LOBO)(131)	Assess long term outcomes in OEF/OIF veterans with combat burn injury, combat nonburn injury, and in civilian burn patients	Secondary	Study design: Prospective cohort Sample: OEF/OIF veterans	4
Women Veterans Cohort Study(132)	Assess health care utilization, costs, stress, and satisfaction in OEF/OIF veterans	Secondary	Study design: Prospective cohort Sample: OEF/OIF veterans	4

Pain in Patients with Polytrauma

Title of Project	Main objective(s) of project	Pain-related variable(s) main or secondary outcome?	Study characteristics	KQ
Pain and Emotional Disorders in Veterans with and without Polytrauma(133)	Describe the prevalence, types, and course of pain and psychiatric disorders, as well as functional outcomes, among OEF/OIF vets with and without polytraumatic injuries	Main	Study design: Prospective cohort Sample: 150-200 polytrauma and 300-400 non-polytrauma OEF/OIF veterans	4
Multidiscipline Assessment of Blast Victims for Cognitive Rehabilitation(134)	Determine whether blast exposure is associated with neuropsychological deficits and/or psychiatric disorder and identify contributors to blast-related post-concussive syndrome	Secondary	Study design: Prospective cohort Sample: OEF/OIF veterans	4
Telerehabilitation of OEF/OIF combat wounded with TBI(135)	Provide care coordination and monitor functional and cognitive outcomes of 45 veterans discharged from a VA PRC with TBI; monitor for adverse effects of pain medication	Secondary	Study design: Prospective cohort Sample: OEF/OIF veterans with TBI	4
Predicting Rehabilitation Costs for VA Patients with Traumatic Brain Injury(136)	Compare cost for rehabilitation for veterans with combat TBI to veterans with non-combat TBI; compare utility of measures in predicting costs; examine affect of PTSD on outcomes/costs	Secondary	Study design: Retrospective cohort Sample: OEF/OIF patients with TBI	4
Characterization and Care Coordination of Polytrauma Patients(137)	Study & describe characteristics of polytrauma patients, including cognitive, emotional, physical and overall functional impairment	Secondary	Study design: Cross-sectional Population: OIF/OEF patients	4
Pain, mental health, and daily function in OIF/OEF veterans(138)	Describe the pain concerns of OIF/OEF veterans, examine association between pain, comorbid mental health concerns, and daily functioning	Main	Study design: Cross-sectional Sample: 233 OIF/OEF veterans	4
Clinical Characteristics of Patients with Polytrauma and Blast-Related Injuries(139)	Describe clinical characteristics, interventions and outcomes for inpatients with polytrauma and blast-related injuries *(Assessment and treatment = primary)*	Main	Study design: Cross-sectional Sample: Veteran inpatients at 4 PRCs	4
Evaluation of Polytrauma Pain(140)	Retrospectively examine pain experiences of soldiers and veterans with polytraumatic injuries incurred during OIF/OEF	Primary	Study design: Cross-sectional Sample: OIF/OEF veterans	4
Validity and reliability of proton magnetic resonance spectroscopy as a diagnostic and outcome measure in clinical trials involving people with SCI(141)	Determine the validity and reliability of Magnetic Resonance Spectroscopy (MRS) as a diagnostic and outcome measure for clinical trials of SCI chronic pain populations; to improve the management of chronic neuropathic pain following SCI	Secondary	Study design: Measurement study Sample: 60 persons with SCI and chronic neuropathic pain, 25 persons with SCI without neuropathic pain, and 25 healthy controls	4

One study is addressing assessment of pain in cognitively impaired patients due to TBI (Key Question 1) using a prospective randomized measurement study of four pain intensity scales in persons with polytrauma and cognitive impairment.(124) Another study will evaluate the usability and utility of CPRS pain assessment templates in two PRC sites; a template contains a module designed to assist clinicians in evaluating pain in patients with cognitive impairment.(125)

Four studies are testing interventions in patients with polytrauma (Key Question 2): Bair is using an RCT design to test a stepped care intervention for OEF/OIF veterans with chronic and disabling musculoskeletal pain.(126) It is expected that some enrollees will meet criteria for polytrauma. Gallagher's prospective cohort study will evaluate the efficacy of early advanced regional anesthetic techniques on pain and mental health outcomes two years post-injury.(128) Using a pre-post evaluation design, Gironda is piloting a brief cognitive headache management intervention for OEF/OIF veterans suffering from persistent blast-related headache.(129) In a controlled clinical trial, Roy is testing whether the Virtual Reality Exposure Therapy and Imaging intervention improves measures of functional health and disability compared to prolonged exposure therapy among veterans with PTSD and TBI.(127)

One study is examining clinical characteristics of headache conditions among OEF/OIF veterans referred to a VA Blast Injury Clinic (Key Question 3).(129)
Thirteen studies will provide information about patient factors associated with outcomes in polytrauma patients (Kew Question 4). Six studies utilizing prospective cohort designs (128, 131-135) and one study using a retrospective cohort design (136) will follow samples of OEF/OIF soldiers or OEF/OIF veterans over time; outcomes include measures of pain, functional status, or adverse effects of pain treatments. Two clinical trials (126, 127) and 5 cross-sectional studies (130, 137-140) will also generate information regarding the relationship of patient factors to pain outcomes in polytrauma patients. An additional study is likely to include polytrauma patients and will examine the validity and reliability of Magnetic Resonance Spectroscopy as a diagnostic tool for clinical trials involving SCI patients with chronic pain.(141) A study objective is to determine pathophysiological and psychosocial contributors to pain after SCI.

Finally, in an ongoing study using qualitative and quantitative methods to evaluate the utility of CPRS pain assessment tools, information will be generated regarding provider or system barriers to treating pain among polytrauma patients (Key Question 5).(125)

Limitations—Active Research

Although we made efforts to identify VA and non-VA investigators who are conducting or planning projects that address key questions, it is very likely that potentially relevant projects were not found. Our primary means of surveying was using email; many investigators did not respond to our queries, and we presume that in many of these cases, these investigators were not doing research relevant to the key questions. A snowball approach was used to identify relevant research projects; this approach identified several of the projects included in this review. We note that we communicated with several military/DOD and a number of non-VA, non-DOD investigators during the process. In addition, we searched a number of web-databases to identify funded VA and non-VA projects.

SUMMARY AND DISCUSSION

Pain from polytraumatic injuries poses numerous challenges during and after rehabilitation treatment. Pain assessment and intervention efforts are further complicated when the injuries include TBI. The overall purpose of this project was to identify and synthesize evidence on the assessment and treatment of pain in polytrauma patients.

Overall, the literature provides very limited evidence to guide clinicians in this area. Although some previous investigations indicate that pain may interfere with neurocognitive performance in TBI patients, there have been no published studies examining approaches to assessing pain among patients with moderate to severe TBI. Studies that have been done with patients with cognitive impairment due to dementia indicate that most cognitively impaired individuals can understand at least one self-assessment measure. Guidelines suggest that for patients with dementia who cannot understand any of several self-assessment measures available, an observational assessment measure or input from family, friends, or staff who know patients well, or empiric pain treatment if the patient has diagnoses usually associated with pain, may be helpful. How well these findings and guidelines might apply to younger patients with cognitive impairment due to TBI is currently unknown. One ongoing VA research study is examining the validity and reliability of 4 pain intensity scales in persons with polytrauma and cognitive impairment, and an additional VA study is examining the utility of a CPRS pain assessment template module to assist clinicians in evaluating pain in patients with cognitive impairment in PRCs.

The literature also provides very limited evidence to guide clinicians in selecting among non-surgical pain treatments in patients with polytrauma. Aside from one good quality retrospective cohort study indicating that rehabilitation may improve outcomes among patients with trauma related amputation, no systematic pain intervention studies have been done in the polytrauma population. A number of case reports suggest possible approaches to treating pain in polytrauma patients, ranging from intrathecal baclofen pumps for pain associated with spasticity to alternative therapies including healing touch. These potential treatment modalities have not been rigorously tested with polytrauma patients. Despite potential concerns about adverse effects, we found only a single case report regarding the use of opioids for pain other than for acute care among TBI patients. Several ongoing research projects are testing interventions in patients with polytrauma. These interventions include stepped care for chronic musculoskeletal pain, advanced regional anesthetic techniques, brief cognitive headache management therapy for persistent blast-related headache, and Virtual Reality Exposure Therapy and Imaging for veterans with PTSD and TBI.

Although several studies show that headache (as well as auditory deficits and otalgia) is common among blast injury patients, there are no published studies describing how blast-related headache might differ in terms of phenomenology or treatment from other types of headache pain. One VA study is currently examining clinical characteristics of headache conditions among OEF/OIF veterans referred to a VA Blast Injury Clinic.

Pain in Patients with Polytrauma

From a number of cohort studies, there is moderate evidence showing that injury factors (including location, severity, and the number of different injuries) are associated with pain and functional status over time. TBI itself is associated with worse outcomes when compared to polytrauma patients without TBI, and there is some evidence that pain is common among TBI patients, present in one-third to one-half of patients up to five years post-injury. However, contrary to what is often reported in the literature and reported in a recent systematic review, we found very limited evidence to support that patients with mild TBI are more likely to have headache or other pain than patients without TBI. While predominantly cross-sectional studies suggest that patients with mild TBI may be more likely to have headache pain than patients with moderate or severe TBI, six prospective cohort studies and several additional cross-sectional studies did not find a relationship between TBI severity and headache prevalence. Most of the cross-sectional studies were done in outpatient settings up to several years post-injury, and did not adjust for potential confounders that may influence relationships between TBI severity and pain. In these studies, cases were identified based on who was referred or attended outpatient follow-up visits. It is thus likely that differences in sample composition contribute to the differences in findings between the cross-sectional and cohort studies, in that patients with mild TBI may be more likely to be referred to or attend outpatient follow-up appointments when they have bothersome or persistent symptoms such as headache.

Overall, we found limited evidence regarding other patient characteristics that are associated with pain-related outcomes in polytrauma patients. Factors found to be associated with worse outcomes across at least several studies were: multiplicity of injury, head injury or cognitive disability, and lower limb injuries. Factors associated with better outcomes in a few studies were: younger age, higher educational achievement, and having a white collar job. Among TBI patients, factors found to be associated with pain and pain-related function in several studies included depression, PTSD, insomnia, and fatigue. Fifteen ongoing research studies will provide additional information about patient factors associated with outcomes in polytrauma patients. Seven studies utilizing cohort designs will follow samples of OEF/OIF soldiers or OEF/OIF veterans over time, and should help to identify important correlates of pain-related outcomes among polytrauma patients.

Finally, there is almost no evidence that addresses provider and system barriers to treatment of pain among polytrauma patients. In one rigorously conducted qualitative study, providers reported that polytrauma patients are very complex to treat, and that the work with this population is very challenging and emotionally taxing. In order to provide high quality care to this complex patient population, clinicians have increased their use of multidisciplinary and concurrent care, and consultation from experts. One active study, which is using qualitative and quantitative methods to evaluate the utility of CPRS pain assessment tools, is likely to generate information regarding provider or system barriers to treating pain among polytrauma patients.

Pain in Patients with Polytrauma

CONCLUSIONS

Table 3. Summary of Systematic Evidence Review by Key Question

Key Question	Type of Evidence	Quality (GRADE) of Evidence*	Comments
1. Are pain assessment tools reliable and valid in patients with cognitive deficits due to TBI?	No direct evidence on pain assessment tools in TBI	Very Low*	■ No particular assessment tool or strategy is known to reliably or validly measure pain intensity or pain-related function in patients with cognitive deficits due to TBI. ■ Most patients with mild cognitive impairment due to dementia can understand at least one pain self-assessment measure. ■ Pain may interfere with neurocognitive functioning in TBI patients. ■ There is no evidence that pain assessment tools for dementia can be reliably applied to persons with cognitive impairment related to TBI
2a. Which treatment approaches are most effective in improving pain outcomes in polytrauma patients?	No direct evidence on effective pain treatment approaches for polytrauma	Very Low	■ No rigorous studies have been done assessing potential benefits or risks of opioids in patients with polytrauma.
2b. Which pain treatment approaches enhance overall rehabilitation efforts?	1 retrospective cohort study	Very Low	■ Inpatient rehabilitation may be associated with increased likelihood of return to work and decreased likelihood of reduced hours of work.
3a. Does blast-related headache pain differ from other types of headache pain?	No evidence comparing blast-related headache to other types of headache	Very Low	■ It is not known how blast-related headache differs from other types of headache in terms of phenomenology or outcome. ■ Headache and auditory deficits are common among patients with blast-injuries.
3b. Which treatments are best for persistent blast-related headache pain?	No evidence on treatment of blast-related headache	---	■ Specific treatments for blast-related related headache pain have not been studied.

Pain in Patients with Polytrauma

Table 3. Summary of Systematic Evidence Review by Key Question, continued

Key Question	Type of Evidence	Quality (GRADE) of Evidence	Comments
4. What patient factors are associated with better and worse clinical outcomes among polytrauma patients? Have interventions been developed to address these factors?	Patients with TBI: 1 systematic review, 10 cohort, 3 case-control, and 11 cross-sectional studies	Very Low	▪ There are mixed findings regarding the association between severity of TBI and pain.
		Low†	▪ Psychological factors, including depression and posttraumatic stress disorder (PTSD), and insomnia and fatigue are associated with pain in TBI patients.
	Other patients: 32 cohort studies, 3 cross-sectional studies	Low	▪ Specific factors associated with worse pain-related outcomes include: multiple injuries, foot injuries or injuries below the knee joint, and concurrent head injury or cognitive disability.
		Very Low	▪ Factors associated with better outcomes are younger age, higher educational achievement, having a white collar job or higher income.
5. What are unique provider and system barriers to detecting and treating pain among polytrauma patients? Have interventions been developed to address these barriers?	1 qualitative study of interviews with providers	Very Low	▪ In qualitative interviews, providers reported that polytrauma patients are very complex to treat, and that the work with this population is very challenging and emotionally taxing. Increasing use of multidisciplinary and concurrent care and consultation from experts may be necessary to provide the care that is needed.

* GRADE: Very low = any estimate of effect is very uncertain.

† GRADE: Low = research is very likely to have an important impact on our confidence in the estimate of effect and may change the effect

FUTURE RESEARCH RECOMMENDATIONS

In order to highlight gaps between the key questions and information available from the literature and information to become available based on current research, Table 4 depicts the results of the literature review of studies that have been published to date, the types of studies necessary to address the key questions, and the research we identified that is currently being done to address the key questions.

Table 5 lists potential study topics and designs as suggested by the investigators and expert reviewers based on the above identified information gaps, and includes their cumulative ratings of the priority of conducting particular studies. Raters were asked to review the research topics and assign them high, medium or low priority, the most important criterion being to achieve the highest possible impact on patient care in the VHA. In rating the suggestions for future research, raters were also asked to consider: 1) the degree to which the proposed research will address information gaps identified in the systematic review, 2) the quantity and quality of the research completed so far including systematic reviews; 3) research currently planned or in progress; 4) the feasibility and timeframe that would be necessary to complete the proposed research; 5) existing barriers that have prevented this research from being undertaken before, and 6) the pros and cons of different research methods that might be appropriate for each research question. Table 5 presents the mean priority ranking for each research topic, based on input from 11 reviewers. Because these are preliminary rankings, a panel or other mechanism to achieve consensus is needed to refine and finalize the recommendations for future research.

We also note the following considerations for conducting and funding research in this area:

- Substantial heterogeneity in the causes and types of polytraumatic injuries, as well as the dynamic nature of recovery from injuries, create challenges for defining and comparing distinct patient populations in research studies, as well as for developing and testing generalizable interventions. In future research it is critical that investigators comprehensively describe polytrauma study samples, settings, recruitment methods, and measurements.
- Due to the level of heterogeneity in the causes and types of polytraumatic injuries, interventions that have the potential to apply, and that are able to be tested among patients with a wide-spectrum of injury patterns may be especially desirable.
- Pilot studies of interventions may be especially helpful to determine feasibility of treatment approaches in the polytrauma patient population before proceeding to larger-scale randomized clinical trials. Enhancement of funding mechanisms that facilitate such pilot work is desirable.
- Battlefield, acute-phase, or early rehabilitation pain interventions may have an important impact on subsequent pain-related outcomes. The DOD may obtain follow-up survey data that could be used or augmented to conduct pain outcome research. Mechanisms that foster improved DOD/VA collaborations including additional data collection may highly desirable. Establishment of a joint DOD-VA pain workgroup might facilitate such collaboration.

Pain in Patients with Polytrauma

Table 4. Summary of Literature Review Findings and Identified Ongoing Research

Key Question or Subquestion	Results of Literature Review	Types of studies needed to answer question	Identified ongoing research
1. Are pain assessment tools reliable and valid in patients with cognitive deficits due to TBI?	No direct evidence on pain assessment tools in TBI or polytrauma.	Qualitative research in rehabilitation patients with polytrauma	▪ Qualitative/quantitative study of clinicians from PRCs regarding pain education & assessment tools(125)
		Prospective observational study of reliability and validity of instruments in rehabilitation patients with polytrauma	▪ Prospective randomized study comparing validity of 4 pain scales in TBI patients(124)
2a. Which treatments improve pain outcomes in polytrauma patients? 2b. Which pain treatment approaches enhance overall rehabilitation efforts?	▪ Case series and case reports of various pain treatments. ▪ Little to no information on use of opioids or integrated care approaches	Exploratory research: feasibility of treatment modalities in case series	▪ Case series pilot of cognitive behavioral intervention for blast headache(129) ▪ Clinical trial of Virtual reality therapy for TBI (pain secondary outcome)(127)
		Effectiveness research: Controlled comparisons of different treatment strategies in patients with polytrauma before or at inception of rehabilitation	▪ RCT of stepped care in OIF/OEF veterans with severe chronic musculoskeletal pain(126) ▪ Prospective cohort study of outcomes of regional anesthesia(128)
3a. Does blast-related headache pain differ from other types of headache pain?	▪ None. ▪ Headache and auditory deficits are common in patients exposed to blast	Prospective, observational studies to determine whether features of injuries, including exposure to blasts, are associated with a different clinical course and outcome.	▪ Case series pilot of cognitive behavioral intervention for blast headache(129)
3b. Which treatments are best for persistent blast-related headache pain?	None.	Exploratory research: feasibility of treatment modalities in case series	▪ Case series on brief cognitive-behavioral headache management treatment (BCBHMT) of blast-TBI((129)
		Effectiveness research: Controlled comparisons of different treatment strategies in patients with blast-related headache	No identified studies using this design

Pain in Patients with Polytrauma

Key Question or Subquestion	Results of Literature Review	Types of studies needed to answer question	Identified ongoing research
4a. What patient factors are associated with better and worse (pain-related) clinical outcomes among polytrauma patients?	■ Cohort, case control, and cross-sectional studies. ■ Injury characteristics, insomnia, fatigue, and psychosocial factors are associated with pain-related outcomes (Grade: Low)	Prospective observational study of factors associated with pain-related outcomes among polytrauma patients. Effectiveness research: Controlled comparisons of different treatment strategies in patients with and without certain characteristics	■ 6 prospective cohort studies examining various (including pain-related) outcomes).(128, 131-135) ■ 1 retrospective cohort study(136) and 5 cross-sectional studies.(130, 137-140) ■ Clinical trial of Virtual reality therapy in TBI patients (pain secondary outcome)(127) ■ RCT of stepped care in OIF/OEF veterans with severe chronic musculoskeletal pain(126)
4b. Have interventions been developed to specifically address these factors?	None.	Exploratory research: feasibility of treatment modalities in case series Effectiveness research: Controlled comparisons of treatment strategies in patients with comorbid conditions	No identified studies using this design No identified studies using this design
5a. What are unique provider and system barriers to detecting and treating pain among polytrauma patients?	One qualitative study of interviews with providers.	Qualitative research in rehabilitation patients with polytrauma Prospective observational study of provider and systems factors associated with pain-related outcomes in polytrauma patients.	■ Qualitative/quantitative study of clinicians from PRCs regarding pain education & assessment tools (125) No identified studies using this design
5b. Have interventions been developed to effectively address these barriers?	None.	Exploratory research: feasibility of treatment modalities in case series Effectiveness research: Controlled comparisons of treatment strategies in patients with polytrauma	No identified studies using this design No identified studies using this design

Pain in Patients with Polytrauma

Table 5: Future Research Topics/Designs – Ratings of Priority

Key Question or Subquestion	Results of Literature Review	Future Research Topic Suggestions	Median rank 1, 2, or 3 1 = most important	Interquartile range
1. Are pain assessment tools reliable and valid in patients with cognitive deficits due to TBI?	No direct evidence on pain assessment tools in TBI or polytrauma.	Quantitative measurement study of reliability and validity of existing pain assessment tools among patients with varying levels of communicativeness and brain injury.	1	1, 2
		Examine the discriminant validity of tools for distinguishing pain from other forms of distress and impairment (e.g., restlessness, PTSD symptoms)	1	1, 2
		Examine the validity of assessment tools in the context of a clinical trial of an intervention for a specific pain condition. For example, in trial of opioids for patients with multiple orthopedic injuries and TBI, use tool to measure changes in pain over time.	2	1, 2
		Examine utility, reliability and validity of CPRS Pain assessment modules being used in VA PRCs for assessment of non-communicative patients with pain.	2	1, 3
		Qualitative study to identify pain behaviors in different cognitively impaired TBI states. From this information, develop and test new tool or modify existing tools to match severity and type of cognitive impairment.	2	1, 3
		Qualitative/quantitative research using partnership with family (and staff) to identify key pain behaviors. Develop or modify tool to incorporate information from patient, caregivers, and empiric trials of analgesics (i.e., guideline recommended approaches).	2	2, 3
2a. Which treatments improve pain outcomes in polytrauma pts?	▪ Primarily case series and case reports of various pain treatments. ▪ Little to no information on use of opioids or integrated care approaches.	Trials of non-pharmacological interventions of varying treatment intensity, including psychological interventions and telephone-based interventions.	1	1, 2
2b. Which pain treatment approaches enhance overall rehab. efforts?		RCTs of integrated treatment approaches including comprehensive interdisciplinary rehab., collaborative care, and treatment involving family members.	1	1, 2
		Compare treatments for common specific core conditions (e.g., TBI; PTSD; Pain) to integrated treatment of these core overlapping symptoms.	1	1, 2
		Systematic prospective observation methods and single case experimental designs with replication to study the relationship between pain control and rehabilitation outcomes.	2	2, 3

Pain in Patients with Polytrauma

Key Question or Subquestion	Results of Literature Review	Future Research Topic Suggestions	Median rank 1, 2, or 3 *1 = most important*	Interquartile range
3a. Does blast-related headache pain differ from other types of headache pain?	• None. • Headache and auditory deficits are common in patients exposed to blast.	Cross sectional study describing and comparing characteristics of veterans with headache presumed to be blast-related to veterans with headache not known to be blast-related.	2	1, 2
		Prospective observational cohort study comparing outcomes of veterans with blast-related headache to those without blast-related headache	2	1, 2
		Study associations between comorbid psychiatric conditions and headache among patients with blast-headache; compare to patients with non-blast-headache	2	1, 2
		Perform routine imaging on soldiers exposed to blast to assess for structural abnormalities and correlate with headache symptoms	2	2, 3
3b. Which treatments are best for persistent blast-related headache pain?	None.	Trials of pharmacologic and non-pharmacologic treatments, including patients with blast-related headache in one arm of the trial. Non-pharmacologic interventions to test include cognitive behavioral treatment, hypnosis, relaxation training, and biofeedback.	1	1, 1
4a. What patient factors are associated with pain-related outcomes in polytrauma patients? Have interventions been developed to specifically address these factors? (see 2. above)	Some evidence that injury characteristics, insomnia, fatigue, and psychosocial factors are associated with pain-related outcomes	Prospective cohort study measuring pain outcomes over time. Measuring contributions of patient characteristics and comorbid conditions, while adjusting for injury characteristics including multiplicity of injury, pain type, and location.	1	1, 2
		Prospective cohort study examining relationships between pain, PTSD, and TBI, and pain-related outcomes	1	1, 2
		Collaborate with DOD to collect or obtain existing pre-deployment DOD survey data to adjust for baseline characteristics prior to injuries in prospective or retrospective cohort studies.	2	2, 2
		Use data obtained in collaboration with DOD and/or from Landsthuhl Regional Medical Center to identify long-term effects of battlefield, acute-phase, or early rehab. treatment.	2	2, 2
		Evaluate contribution of partnership with family and other social variables to pain-related outcomes in polytrauma patients.	2	2, 3

Pain in Patients with Polytrauma

Key Question or Subquestion	Results of Literature Review	Future Research Topic Suggestions	Median rank 1, 2, or 3 1 = most important	Interquartile range
5a. What are unique provider and system barriers to detecting and treating pain among polytrauma patients? Have interventions been developed to effectively address these barriers?	One qualitative study of interviews with providers.	Establish treatment guidelines for pain in polytrauma based on expert opinion. Disseminate and measure impact of guidelines on care.	1	1, 2
		Evaluate patient perceptions of provider and systems barriers, and the impact of efforts to mitigate those barriers.	2	1, 2
		Evaluate implementation of CPRS pain assessment tools in PRCs. Refine tools and reevaluate.	2	1, 2
		Couple evaluation of site-specific organizational factors with multi-site prospective observational study of patient pain-related outcomes. Identify associations between organizational factors and patient outcomes.	2	1, 2
		Identify adaptations PRCs are making to accommodate diversity among polytrauma patients with pain.	2	2, 3
		Measure the impact of polytrauma pain education on provider behavior.	2	2, 3
		Formative evaluation of implementation of guidelines and education and impact on treatment processes in PRCs.	2	2, 3

Pain in Patients with Polytrauma

REFERENCES

1.   Lew HL, Poole JH, Vanderploeg RD, Goodrich GL, Dekelboum S, Guillory SB, et al. Program development and defining characteristics of returning military in a VA Polytrauma Network Site. Journal of rehabilitation research and development 2007;44(7):1027-1034.
2.   Gawande A. Casualties of war--military care for the wounded from Iraq and Afghanistan. New England Journal of Medicine 2004;351(24):2471-5.
3.   Friedemann-Sanchez G, Sayer NA, Pickett T. Provider perspectives on rehabilitation of patients with polytrauma. Archives of Physical Medicine and Rehabilitation 2008;89(1):171-178.
4.   Warden D. Military TBI during the Iraq and Afghanistan wars. Journal of Head Trauma Rehabilitation 2006;21(5):398-402.
5.   Montgomery SP, Swiecki CW, Shriver CD. The evaluation of casualties from Operation Iraqi Freedom on return to the continental United States from March to June 2003. Journal of the American College of Surgeons 2005;201(1):7-12; discussion 12-3.
6.   Lin DL, Kirk KL, Murphy KP, McHale KA, Doukas WC. Evaluation of orthopaedic injuries in Operation Enduring Freedom. Journal of Orthopaedic Trauma 2004;18(8 Suppl):S48-53.
7.   Okie S. Traumatic brain injury in the war zone. New England Journal of Medicine 2005;352(20):2043-7.
8.   Scott SG, Belanger HG, Vanderploeg RD, Massengale J, Scholten J. Mechanism-of-injury approach to evaluating patients with blast-related polytrauma. Journal of the American Osteopathic Association 2006;106(5):265-70.
9.   DePalma RG, Burris DG, Champion HR, Hodgson MJ. Blast injuries. New England Journal of Medicine 2005;352(13):1335-42.
10.   Okie S. Reconstructing lives--a tale of two soldiers. New England Journal of Medicine 2006;355(25):2609-15.
11.   Harris RP, Helfand M, Woolf SH, Lohr KN, Mulrow CD, Teutsch SM, et al. Current methods of the US Preventive Services Task Force: a review of the process. American Journal of Preventive Medicine 2001;20(3 Suppl):21-35.
12.   Atkins D, Best D, Briss PA, Eccles M, Falck-Ytter Y, Flottorp S, et al. Grading quality of evidence and strength of recommendations. BMJ 2004;328(7454):1490.
13.   Nicholson K. Pain, cognition and traumatic brain injury. NeuroRehabilitation 2000;14(2):95-103.
14.   Nicholson K, Martelli MF, Zasler ND. Does pain confound interpretation of neuropsychological test results? Neurorehabilitation 2001;16(4):225-30.
15.   Hart RP, Martelli MF, Zasler ND. Chronic pain and neuropsychological functioning. Neuropsychology Review 2000;10(3):131-49.
16.   Grace GM, Nielson WR, Hopkins M, Berg MA. Concentration and memory deficits in patients with fibromyalgia syndrome. Journal of Clinical & Experimental Neuropsychology: Official Journal of the International Neuropsychological Society 1999;21(4):477-87.
17.   Kewman DG, Vaishampayan N, Zald D, Han B. Cognitive impairment in musculoskeletal pain patients. International Journal of Psychiatry in Medicine 1991;21(3):253-62.

18.   Veiel HO. A preliminary profile of neuropsychological deficits associated with major depression. Journal of Clinical & Experimental Neuropsychology: Official Journal of the International Neuropsychological Society 1997;19(4):587-603.

19.   Eccleston C, Crombez G, Aldrich S, Stannard C. Attention and somatic awareness in chronic pain. Pain 1997;72(1-2):209-15.

20.   Pilcher JJ, Huffcutt AI. Effects of sleep deprivation on performance: a meta-analysis. Sleep 1996;19(4):318-26.

21.   Helfand M, Freeman M. Assessment and management of acute pain in adult medical inpatients: A systematic review. Washington, DC 2007.

22.   Herr K, Bjoro K, Decker S. Tools for assessment of pain in nonverbal older adults with dementia: a state-of-the-science review. Journal of Pain & Symptom Management 2006;31(2):170-92.

23.   van Herk R, van Dijk M, Baar FP, Tibboel D, de Wit R. Observation scales for pain assessment in older adults with cognitive impairments or communication difficulties. Nurs Res 2007;56(1):34-43.

24.   Zwakhalen SMG, Hamers JPH, Abu-Saad HH, Berger MPF. Pain in elderly people with severe dementia: a systematic review of behavioural pain assessment tools. BMC Geriatrics 2006;6:3.

25.   Stolee P, Hillier LM, Esbaugh J, Bol N, McKellar L, Gauthier N. Instruments for the assessment of pain in older persons with cognitive impairment. Journal of the American Geriatrics Society 2005;53(2):319-26.

26.   Hadjistavropoulos T, Herr K, Turk DC, Fine PG, Dworkin RHP, Helme RM, PhD [P], et al. An Interdisciplinary Expert Consensus Statement on Assessment of Pain in Older Persons. Clinical Journal of Pain 2007;23 Supplement 1:S1-S43.

27.   Fuchs-Lacelle S, Hadjistavropoulos T. Development and preliminary validation of the pain assessment checklist for seniors with limited ability to communicate (PACSLAC). Pain Management Nursing 2004;5(1):37-49.

28.   Warden V, Hurley AC, Volicer L. Development and psychometric evaluation of the Pain Assessment in Advanced Dementia (PAINAD) scale. In: Journal of the American Medical Directors Association; 2003. p. 9-15.

29.   Parmelee P. Pain complaints and cognitive status among elderly institution residents. Journal of the American Geriatrics Society 1993;41(5):517-522.

30.   Pautex S, Michon A, Guedira M, Emond H, Le Lous P, Samaras D, et al. Pain in severe dementia: self-assessment or observational scales?. Journal of the American Geriatrics Society 2006;54(7):1040-5.

31.   Buffum MD, Hutt E, Chang VT, Craine MH, Snow AL. Cognitive impairment and pain management: Review of issues and challenges. Journal of Rehabilitation Research & Development 2007;44(2):315-30.

32.   Anonymous. Assessing Pain in the Patient with Impaired Communication: A Consensus Statement from the VHA National Pain Management Strategy Coordinating Committee. In: Affairs V, editor.; 2004.

33.   Pezzin LE, Dillingham TR, MacKenzie EJ. Rehabilitation and the long-term outcomes of persons with trauma-related amputations. Archives of Physical Medicine & Rehabilitation 2000;81(3):292-300.

34.   Hassantash SA, Afrakhteh M, Maier RV. Causalgia: a meta-analysis of the literature. Archives of Surgery 2003;138(11):1226-31.

35.   Andy OJ. Post concussion syndrome: brainstem seizures, a case report. Clinical Electroencephalography 1989;20(1):24-34.

36.   Donnellan CP. Acupuncture for central pain affecting the ribcage following traumatic brain injury and rib fractures--a case report. Acupuncture in Medicine 2006;24(3):129-33.

37.   Bergfeldt U, Borg K, Kullander K, Julin P. Focal spasticity therapy with botulinum toxin: effects on function, activities of daily living and pain in 100 adult patients. Journal of Rehabilitation Medicine 2006;38(3):166-71.

38.   Ribbers GM, Stam HJ. Complex regional pain syndrome type I treated with topical capsaicin: a case report. Archives of Physical Medicine and Rehabilitation 2001;82(6):851-852.

39.   Zachariah SB, Borges EF, Varghese R, Cruz AR, Ross GS. Positive response to oral divalproex sodium (Depakote) in patients with spasticity and pain. American Journal of the Medical Sciences 1994;308(1):38-40.

40.   Adeloye A. Clinical trial of fluphenazine in the post-concussional syndrome. Practitioner 1971;206(234):517-9.

41.   Childers MK, Holland D. Psychomotor agitation following gabapentin use in brain injury. Brain Injury 1997;11(7):537-40.

42.   Batten SV, Pollack SJ. Integrative outpatient treatment for returning service members. J Clin Psychol 2008;64(8):928-39.

43.   Wardell DW, Rintala DH, Duan Z, Tan G. A pilot study of healing touch and progressive relaxation for chronic neuropathic pain in persons with spinal cord injury. Journal of Holistic Nursing 2006;24(4):231-40; discussion 241-4.

44.   Jang SH, Shin SW, Ahn SH, Cho IH, Kim SH. Radiation therapy for heterotopic ossification in a patient with traumatic brain injury. Yonsei Medical Journal 2000;41(4):536-9.

45.   Denys P, Azouvi P, Denormandie P, Samuel C, Patel A, Bussel B. Late cognitive and behavioural improvement following treatment of disabling orthopaedic complications of a severe closed head injury. Brain Injury 1996;10(2):149-53.

46.   Concalves J, Garcia-March G, Sanchez-Ledesma MJ, Onzain I, Broseta J. Management of intractable spasticity of supraspinal origin by chronic cervical intrathecal infusion of baclofen. Stereotactic & Functional Neurosurgery 1994;62(1-4):108-12.

47.   Broseta J, Garcia-March G, Sanchez-Ledesma MJ, Anaya J, Silva I. Chronic intrathecal baclofen administration in severe spasticity. Stereotactic & Functional Neurosurgery 1990;54-55:147-53.

48.   Becker R, Alberti O, Bauer BL. Continuous intrathecal baclofen infusion in severe spasticity after traumatic or hypoxic brain injury. Journal of Neurology 1997;244(3):160-6.

49.   Francisco GE, Hu MM, Boake C, Ivanhoe CB. Efficacy of early use of intrathecal baclofen therapy for treating spastic hypertonia due to acquired brain injury. Brain Injury 2005;19(5):359-64.

50.   Francisco GE, Latorre JM, Ivanhoe CB. Intrathecal baclofen therapy for spastic hypertonia in chronic traumatic brain injury. Brain Injury 2007;21(3):335-8.

51.   Son BC, Lee SW, Choi ES, Sung JH, Hong JT. Motor cortex stimulation for central pain following a traumatic brain injury. Pain 2006;123(1-2):210-6.

52.   Gallagher R, Drance E, Higginbotham S. Finding the person behind the pain: chronic pain management in a patient with traumatic brain injury. Journal of the American Medical Directors Association 2006;7(7):432-4.

53.   Chen KW, Turner FD. A case study of simultaneous recovery from multiple physical symptoms with medical qigong therapy. Journal of Alternative & Complementary Medicine 2004;10(1):159-62.

54.   Shah RV, Racz GB. Long-term relief of posttraumatic headache by sphenopalatine ganglion pulsed radiofrequency lesioning: a case report. Archives of Physical Medicine & Rehabilitation 2004;85(6):1013-6.

55.   Verdolin MH, Stedje-Larsen ET, Hickey AH. Ten consecutive cases of complex regional pain syndrome of less than 12 months duration in active duty United States military personnel treated with spinal cord stimulation. Anesth Analg 2007;104(6):1557-60, table of contents.

56.   Leyton N. Post-concussional migraine: a successful response to treatment. The Medical press 1951;226(2):46-47.

57.   Hoge CW, McGurk D, Thomas JL, Cox AL, Engel CC, Castro CA. Mild traumatic brain injury in U.S. Soldiers returning from Iraq. N Engl J Med 2008;358(5):453-63.

58.   Warden DL, Ryan LM, Helmick KM, Schwab K, French L, Lu W, et al. War Neurotrauma: the Defense and Veterans Brain Injury Center (DVBIC) Experience at Walter Reed Army Medical Center (WRAMC). In: The 23rd Annual National Neurotrauma Society Symposium; 2005 November 10-11, 2005; Washington, DC; 2005.

59.   Cernak IMDP, Savic JMDP, Ignjatovic DMDP, Jevtic MMDP. Blast Injury from Explosive Munitions. Journal of Trauma-Injury Infection & Critical Care 1999;47(1):96-103.

60.   Cave KM, Cornish EM, Chandler DW. Blast injury of the ear: clinical update from the global war on terror. Military Medicine 2007;172(7):726-30.

61.   Taher AA, Johns RM. Mandibular joint dysfunction otalgia caused by a bomb explosion wave. Journal of Craniofacial Surgery 1992;3(4):223-5.

62.   Lew HL, Lin P-H, Fuh J-L, Wang S-J, Clark DJ, Walker WC. Characteristics and treatment of headache after traumatic brain injury: a focused review. American Journal of Physical Medicine & Rehabilitation 2006;85(7):619-27.

63.   Baandrup L, Jensen R. Chronic post-traumatic headache--a clinical analysis in relation to the International Headache Classification 2nd Edition. Cephalalgia 2005;25(2):132-8.

64.   Bekkelund SI, Salvesen R. Prevalence of head trauma in patients with difficult headache: the North Norway Headache Study. Headache 2003;43(1):59-62.

65.   Bettucci D, Aguggia M, Bolamperti L, Riccio A, Mutani R. Chronic post-traumatic headache associated with minor cranial trauma: a description of cephalalgic patterns. Italian Journal of Neurological Sciences 1998;19(1):20-4.

66.   Haas DC. Characteristics of chronic posttraumatic headache. Headache 2002;42(2):162-3.

67.   Radanov BP, Di Stefano G, Augustiny KF. Symptomatic approach to posttraumatic headache and its possible implications for treatment. European Spine Journal 2001;10(5):403-7.

68.   Nampiaparampil DE. Prevalence of chronic pain after traumatic brain injury: a systematic review. JAMA 2008;300(6):711-9.

69.   Schaller WF. After-effects of Head Injury. The Journal of the American Medical Association 1939;113(20):1779-1785.

70.   Walker WC, Seel RT, Curtiss G, Warden DL. Headache after moderate and severe traumatic brain injury: a longitudinal analysis. Archives of Physical Medicine & Rehabilitation 2005;86(9):1793-800.

71.   Hoffman JM, Pagulayan KF, Zawaideh N, Dikmen S, Temkin N, Bell KR. Understanding pain after traumatic brain injury: impact on community participation. American Journal of Physical Medicine & Rehabilitation 2007;86(12):962-9.

72.   Bryant RA, Marosszeky JE, Crooks J, Baguley IJ, Gurka JA. Interaction of posttraumatic stress disorder and chronic pain following traumatic brain injury. Journal of Head Trauma Rehabilitation 1999;14(6):588-94.

73.   Masson F, Maurette P, Salmi LR, Dartigues JF, Vecsey J, Destaillats JM, et al. Prevalence of impairments 5 years after a head injury, and their relationship with disabilities and outcome. Brain Injury 1996;10(7):487-97.

74.   Hillier SL, Sharpe MH, Metzer J. Outcomes 5 years post-traumatic brain injury (with further reference to neurophysical impairment and disability). Brain Injury 1997;11(9):661-75.

75.   Guttman E. Postcontusional Headache. Lancet 1943;1:10-12.

76.   Olver JH, Ponsford JL, Curran CA. Outcome following traumatic brain injury: a comparison between 2 and 5 years after injury. Brain Injury 1996;10(11):841-8.

77.   Cosgrove JL, Vargo M, Reidy ME. A prospective study of peripheral nerve lesions occurring in traumatic brain-injured patients. American Journal of Physical Medicine & Rehabilitation 1989;68(1):15-7.

78.   Cantor JB, Ashman T, Gordon W, Ginsberg A, Engmann C, Egan M, et al. Fatigue after traumatic brain injury and its impact on participation and quality of life. The Journal of head trauma rehabilitation 2008;23(1):41-51.

79.   Beetar JT, Guilmette TJ, Sparadeo FR. Sleep and pain complaints in symptomatic traumatic brain injury and neurologic populations. Archives of Physical Medicine & Rehabilitation 1996;77(12):1298-302.

80.   Sayer NA, Chiros CE, Sigford B, Scott S, Clothier B, Pickett T, et al. Characteristics and rehabilitation outcomes among patients with blast and other injuries sustained during the Global War on Terror. Archives of Physical Medicine and Rehabilitation 2008;89(1):163-170.

81.   Lahz S, Bryant RA. Incidence of chronic pain following traumatic brain injury. Archives of Physical Medicine & Rehabilitation 1996;77(9):889-91.

82.   Wilkinson M, Gilchrist E. Post-traumatic headache. Upsala Journal of Medical Sciences - Supplement 1980;31:48-51.

83.   Leung J, Moseley A, Fereday S, Jones T, Fairbairn T, Wyndham S. The prevalence and characteristics of shoulder pain after traumatic brain injury. Clinical Rehabilitation 2007;21(2):171-81.

84.   Gellman H, Keenan MA, Stone L, Hardy SE, Waters RL, Stewart C. Reflex sympathetic dystrophy in brain-injured patients. Pain 1992;51(3):307-11.

85.   Uomoto JM, Esselman PC. Traumatic brain injury and chronic pain: differential types and rates by head injury severity. Archives of Physical Medicine & Rehabilitation 1993;74(1):61-4.

86.   Yamaguchi M. Incidence of headache and severity of head injury. Headache 1992;32(9):427-31.

87.   Brenner C. Post-traumatic headache. J Neurosurgery 1944;1:379--391.

88.   Russell WR. Cerebral involvement in head injury: a study based on the examination of two hundred cases. Brain 1932;55:549-562.

89.   MacKenzie EJ, McCarthy ML, Ditunno JF, Forrester-Staz C, Gruen GS, Marion DW, et al. Using the SF-36 for characterizing outcome after multiple trauma involving head injury. J Trauma 2002;52(3):527-34.

90.   Ulvik A, Kvale R, Wentzel-Larsen T, Flaatten H. Quality of life 2-7 years after major trauma. Acta Anaesthesiologica Scandinavica 2008;52(2):195-201.

91.   Couch JR, Bearss C. Chronic daily headache in the posttrauma syndrome: relation to extent of head injury. Headache 2001;41(6):559-64.

92.   Kay DW, Kerr TA, Lassman LP. Brain trauma and the postconcussional syndrome. Lancet 1971;2(7733):1052-5.

93.   Tsushima WT, Tsushima VG. Relation between headaches and neuropsychological functioning among head injury patients. Headache 1993;33(3):139-42.

94.   Bay E, Donders J. Risk factors for depressive symptoms after mild-to-moderate traumatic brain injury. Brain Inj 2008;22(3):233-41.

95.   Bushnik T, Englander J, Katznelson L. Fatigue after TBI: association with neuroendocrine abnormalities. Brain Inj 2007;21(6):559-66.

96.   Ouellet M-C, Beaulieu-Bonneau S, Morin CM. Insomnia in patients with traumatic brain injury: frequency, characteristics, and risk factors. Journal of Head Trauma Rehabilitation 2006;21(3):199-212.

97.   Fichtenberg NL, Millis SR, Mann NR, Zafonte RD, Millard AE. Factors associated with insomnia among post-acute traumatic brain injury survivors. Brain Injury 2000;14(7):659-67.

98.   Roganovic Z, Mandic-Gajic G. Pain syndromes after missile-caused peripheral nerve lesions: part 2--treatment. Neurosurgery 2006;59(6):1238-49; discussion 1249-51.

99.   Roganovic Z, Mandic-Gajic G. Pain syndromes after missile-caused peripheral nerve lesions: part 1--clinical characteristics. Neurosurgery 2006;59(6):1226-36; discussion 1236-7.

100.   Frink M, Klaus A-K, Kuther G, Probst C, Gosling T, Kobbe P, et al. Long term results of compartment syndrome of the lower limb in polytraumatised patients. Injury 2007;38(5):607-13.

101.   Dougherty PJ. Transtibial amputees from the Vietnam War. Twenty-eight-year follow-up. Journal of Bone & Joint Surgery - American Volume 2001;83-A(3):383-9.

102.   Dougherty PJ. Long-term follow-up study of bilateral above-the-knee amputees from the Vietnam War. Journal of Bone & Joint Surgery - American Volume 1999;81(10):1384-90.

103.   Lacoux PA, Crombie IK, Macrae WA. Pain in traumatic upper limb amputees in Sierra Leone. Pain 2002;99(1-2):309-12.

104.   Millstein S, Bain D, Hunter GA. A review of employment patterns of industrial amputees--factors influencing rehabilitation. Prosthetics & Orthotics International 1985;9(2):69-78.

105.   Zelle BA, Brown SR, Panzica M, Lohse R, Sittaro NA, Krettek C, et al. The impact of injuries below the knee joint on the long-term functional outcome following polytrauma. Injury 2005;36(1):169-77.

106.   Tran T, Thordarson D. Functional outcome of multiply injured patients with associated foot injury. Foot & Ankle International 2002;23(4):340-3.

107.   Turchin DC, Schemitsch EH, McKee MD, Waddell JP. Do foot injuries significantly affect the functional outcome of multiply injured patients? Journal of Orthopaedic Trauma 1999;13(1):1-4.

108.   Urquhart DM, Williamson OD, Gabbe BJ, Cicuttini FM, Cameron PA, Richardson MD, et al. Outcomes of patients with orthopaedic trauma admitted to level 1 trauma centres. ANZ Journal of Surgery 2006;76(7):600-6.

109.   Brenneman FD, Katyal D, Boulanger BR, Tile M, Redelmeier DA. Long-term outcomes in open pelvic fractures. Journal of Trauma-Injury Infection & Critical Care 1997;42(5):773-7.

110.   Hebert JS, Burnham RS. The effect of polytrauma in persons with traumatic spine injury. A prospective database of spine fractures. Spine 2000;25(1):55-60.

111.   Vles WJ, Steyerberg EW, Essink-Bot ML, van Beeck EF, Meeuwis JD, Leenen LP. Prevalence and determinants of disabilities and return to work after major trauma. J Trauma 2005;58(1):126-35.

112.   Anke AG, Stanghelle JK, Finset A, Roaldsen KS, Pillgram-Larsen J, Fugl-Meyer AR. Long-term prevalence of impairments and disabilities after multiple trauma. Journal of Trauma-Injury Infection & Critical Care 1997;42(1):54-61.

113.   Soberg HL, Bautz-Holter E, Roise O, Finset A. Long-term multidimensional functional consequences of severe multiple injuries two years after trauma: a prospective longitudinal cohort study. Journal of Trauma-Injury Infection & Critical Care 2007;62(2):461-70.

114.   Holtslag HR, van Beeck EF, Lindeman E, Leenen LPH. Determinants of long-term functional consequences after major trauma. Journal of Trauma-Injury Infection & Critical Care 2007;62(4):919-27.

115.   Meerding WJ, Looman CW, Essink-Bot ML, Toet H, Mulder S, van Beeck EF. Distribution and determinants of health and work status in a comprehensive population of injury patients. J Trauma 2004;56(1):150-61.

116.   Mkandawire NC, Boot DA, Braithwaite IJ, Patterson M. Musculoskeletal recovery 5 years after severe injury: long term problems are common. Injury 2002;33(2):111-5.

117.   Dimopoulou I, Anthi A, Mastora Z, Theodorakopoulou M, Konstandinidis A, Evangelou E, et al. Health-related quality of life and disability in survivors of multiple trauma one year after intensive care unit discharge. American Journal of Physical Medicine & Rehabilitation 2004;83(3):171-6.

118.   Brenneman FD, Redelmeier DA, Boulanger BR, McLellan BA, Culhane JP. Long-term outcomes in blunt trauma: who goes back to work? J Trauma 1997;42(5):778-81.

119.   MacKenzie EJ, Morris JA, Jr., Jurkovich GJ, Yasui Y, Cushing BM, Burgess AR, et al. Return to work following injury: the role of economic, social, and job-related factors. Am J Public Health 1998;88(11):1630-7.

120.   Stalp M, Koch C, Ruchholtz S, Regel G, Panzica M, Krettek C, et al. Standardized outcome evaluation after blunt multiple injuries by scoring systems: a clinical follow-up

investigation 2 years after injury. Journal of Trauma-Injury Infection & Critical Care 2002;52(6):1160-8.

121.   Lippert-Gruner M, Maegele M, Haverkamp H, Klug N, Wedekind C. Health-related quality of life during the first year after severe brain trauma with and without polytrauma. Brain Inj 2007;21(5):451-5.

122.   Fitzharris M, Fildes B, Charlton J, Kossmann T. General health status and functional disability following injury in traffic crashes. Traffic Injury Prevention 2007;8(3):309-20.

123.   Taber KH, Warden DL, Hurley RA. Blast-related traumatic brain injury: what is known? Journal of Neuropsychiatry & Clinical Neurosciences 2006;18(2):141-5.

124.   Walker W. Concurrent Validity of Four Pain Intensity Scales in persons with Polytrauma and Cognitive Impairment. A research study in progress. Richmond VAMC.

125.   Kerns R. Pain Assessment in Polytrauma Rehabilitation Centers (PRCs). A research study in progress. HSR&D QUERI Program RRP07-288. VA Connecticut Healthcare System.

126.   Bair M. Evaluation of Stepped CAre for Chronic Pain (ESCAPE). A research study in progress. VA Rehabilitative Research and Development F44371. Indianapolis VAMC.

127.   Roy MJ. The ViRTICo Trial: Virtual Reality Therapy & Imaging in Combat Veterans. A research study in progress. Uniformed Services University, Bethesda MD.

128.   Gallagher RM. Regional Anesthesia Military Battlefield Pain Outcomes Study. A research study in progress. RR&D Service 951. Philadelphia VAMC.

129.   Gironda RJ. Chronic Headache among OEF/OIF Veterans Exposed to Blasts. A research study in progress. Tampa VAMC.

130.   Afari N. Headaches in veterans returning from Iraq/Afghanistan: relation to trauma and combat-related injury. A research study in progress. San Diego VAMC.

131.   Lawrence VA. Long-term Outcomes in Burned OEF/OIF Veterans (LOBO). A research study in progress. VA HSR&D SDR 07-042. San Antonio VAMC.

132.   Brandt C, Haskell S. Women Veterans Cohort Study. A research study in progress. HSR&D DHI 07-065-2. VA Connecticut Healthcare System.

133.   Clark ME. Pain and Emotional Disorders in Veterans with and without Polytrauma. A research study in progress. HSR&D SDR-07-047. Tampa VAMC.

134.   Storzbach D. Multidiscipline Assessment of Blast Victims for Cognitive Rehabilitation. A research study in progress. VHA RR&D B5060R. Portland VAMC.

135.   Siddharthan K. Telerehabilitation of OEF/OIF combat wounded with TBI. A research study in progress. Tampa VAMC.

136.   Lew H. Predicting Rehabilitation Costs for VA Patients with Traumatic Brain Injury. A research study in progress. VA Boston HealthCare System.

137.   Lew H. Characterization and Care Coordination of Polytrauma Patients. A research study in progress. VA Boston HealthCare System.

138.   Helmer D. Pain, mental health, and daily function in OIF/OEF veterans. A research study in progress. Houston VAMC.

139.   Lew H. Clinical Characteristics of Patients with Polytrauma and Blast-Related Injuries. A research study in progress. VA Boston HealthCare System.

140.   Walker RL. Evaluation of Polytrauma Pain. A research study in progress. Tampa VAMC.

141.   Widerstrom-Noga E. Validity and reliability of proton magnetic resonance spectroscopy as a diagnostic and outcome measure in clinical pain trials involving people with spinal cord injury. A research study in progress. Miami VA HCS.

142.   Goel A, Phalke U, Cacciola F, Muzumdar D. Atlantoaxial instability and retroodontoid mass--two case reports. Neurologia Medico-Chirurgica 2004;44(11):603-6.

Pain in Patients with Polytrauma

APPENDIX A. SEARCH STRATEGY

Two librarians (AH and RC) independently designed search strategies based on the key questions. The results of both searches were combined into a single reference library.

Below is the search strategy designed by AH:

Database: Ovid MEDLINE(R) <1950 to January Week 5 2008>
Search Strategy:

```
1    polytraum$.mp. (2115)
2    exp Multiple Trauma/ (7404)
3    (multiple adj3 (wound$ or injur$ or traum$ or casualt$)).mp. (12171)
4    1 or 2 or 3 (13048)
5    exp Blast Injuries/ (1862)
6    exp Brain Injuries/ (34104)
7    ((head or crani$ or cereb$ or brain$ or explosi$ or explod$ or blast$) adj3 (traum$ or wound$ or injur$
or damag$)).mp. (88531)
8    5 or 6 or 7 (90818)
9    exp pain/ (218224)
10   exp pain measurement/ (33373)
11   exp nociceptors/ (8377)
12   (pain$ or agony or agoniz$ or nocicept$).mp. [mp=title, original title, abstract, name of substance
word, subject heading word] (334241)
13   9 or 10 or 11 or 12 (392032)
14   9 or 10 (230078)
15   4 and 14 (175)
16   5 and 14 (12)
17   exp War/ (25443)
18   exp Military Personnel/ (15657)
19   exp Military Medicine/ (21662)
20   exp Veterans/ (5122)
21   exp Veterans Disability Claims/ (209)
22   Hospitals, Veterans/ (4480)
23   exp "United States Department of Veterans Affairs"/ (3021)
24   (desert storm or gulf war or enduring freedom or iraqi freedom).mp. (1606)
25   exp Iraq War, 2003 -/ or exp Iraq/ (2569)
26   (iraq or soldier$ or veteran$ or combat$ or militar$ or battle$).mp. (77729)
27   17 or 18 or 19 or 20 or 21 or 22 or 23 or 24 or 25 or 26 (94873)
28   exp "wounds and injuries"/ or in.fs. (580168)
29   27 and 28 (9834)
30   8 and 13 (1988)
31   limit 30 to humans (1836)
32   limit 31 to english language (1402)
33   limit 31 to abstracts (1447)
34   32 or 33 (1681)
35   4 and 13 (500)
36   limit 35 to humans (491)
37   limit 36 to english language (359)
38   limit 36 to abstracts (465)
39   37 or 38 (483)
40   13 and 29 (449)
```

Pain in Patients with Polytrauma

41   limit 40 to humans (441)
42   limit 41 to english language (383)
43   limit 41 to abstracts (375)
44   42 or 43 (424)
45   34 or 39 or 44 (2480)
46   limit 45 to yr="2000 - 2008" (1163)
47   limit 45 to yr="1902 - 1999" (1317)
48   from 47 keep 1 (1)

Below is the search strategy designed by RC. This search was saved in PubMed to provide automatic weekly updates:

"Brain Injuries"(142)
OR "Multiple Trauma"(142)
OR "Blast Injuries"(142)
OR TBI[All Fields]
OR "traumatic brain injury"[All Fields]
OR "traumatic brain injuries"[All Fields]
OR polytrauma[All Fields]
OR multitrauma[All Fields]
OR "multi trauma"[All Fields]
OR "poly trauma"[All Fields]
OR (("Wounds and Injuries"(142) OR "injuries "[Subheading]) AND ("War"(142) OR "Iraq War, 2003 -"(142)
OR "Gulf War"(142)))
AND ("pain"[MeSH Terms] OR pain[Text Word])

Pain in Patients with Polytrauma

APPENDIX B. ARTICLE SCREENING FORM

Author, Year _____   Title _____

1. Does the study population constitute or include:
  a. Polytrauma patients in or after rehab phase ....❏
  b. Patients with blast-related headaches ....❏
  c. Neither a) nor b) ....STOP
 	
2. Does the study intervention strictly address:
  a. Perioperative or surgical pain management ....STOP
  b. Treatment for burn injuries only ....STOP
 	
3. Do the study outcomes include measures of pain (pain intensity and/or pain-related function)?
  c. No ....STOP
  d. Yes ....❏
	Key words or categories:

4. Is the text of the article in English?
  a. No ....STOP
  b. Yes ....❏
 	
5. Does the article provide primary data?
  a. No (letter/commentary/non-systematic review) ....STOP
  b. Yes ....❏
 	
6. If this article meets no other criterion, should it be saved for background?
  a. No ....STOP
  b. Yes ....❏
	Notes:

Circle the Key Question(s) to which this article applies:

6. Have reliable and valid measures and assessment tools been developed to measure pain intensity and pain-related functional interference among patients with cognitive deficits due to TBI? Which measures and tools are likely to be most useful in assessing pain in polytrauma patients with cognitive deficits due to TBI?

7. Which treatment approaches are most likely to be effective in improving pain outcomes (pain intensity and functional interference) in polytrauma patients? Which pain treatment approaches are most likely to enhance overall rehabilitation efforts?

8. Does blast-related headache pain differ in terms of phenomenology and treatment from other types of headache pain? Which treatments are best for persistent blast-related headache pain?

9. What factors are associated with better and worse clinical outcomes among polytrauma patients? Have interventions been developed to specifically address these factors?

10. What are unique provider and system barriers to detecting and treating pain among polytrauma patients? Have interventions been developed to effectively address these barriers?

For reference: Definition of Polytrauma: Concurrent injury to two or more body parts or systems that results in cognitive, physical, psychological or other psychosocial impairments. Combat-related mental conditions co-occurring with injury to at least one other system also constitutes polytrauma. Scope of Review: The scope includes the assessment and treatment in rehabilitation and post-rehabilitation care settings of persistent pain or exacerbations of pain resulting from polytraumatic injuries. The scope of this review excludes the following: battlefield/emergency assessment and care; treatment of burn injuries; choice of surgical strategy, and perioperative management of injuries suffered in trauma. The scope also excludes post-traumatic/post-concussive headache unrelated to blast injury, unless the sample includes patients with moderate or greater cognitive deficit.

APPENDIX C.   USPSTF QUALITY RATING CRITERIA

Randomized Controlled Trials (RCTs) and Cohort Studies

Criteria

- Initial assembly of comparable groups: RCTs—adequate randomization, including concealment and whether potential confounders were distributed equally among groups; cohort studies—consideration of potential confounders with either restriction or measurement for adjustment in the analysis; consideration of inception cohorts
- Maintenance of comparable groups (includes attrition, cross-overs, adherence, contamination)
- Important differential loss to follow-up or overall high loss to follow-up
- Measurements: equal, reliable, and valid (includes masking of outcome assessment)
- Clear definition of interventions
- Important outcomes considered
- Analysis: adjustment for potential confounders for cohort studies, or intention-to-treat analysis for RCTs (i.e. analysis in which all participants in a trial are analyzed according to the intervention to which they were allocated, regardless of whether or not they completed the intervention)

Definition of ratings based on above criteria

Good: Meets all criteria: Comparable groups are assembled initially and maintained throughout the study (follow-up at least 80 percent); reliable and valid measurement instruments are used and applied equally to the groups; interventions are spelled out clearly; important outcomes are considered; and appropriate attention to confounders in analysis.

Fair: Studies will be graded "fair" if any or all of the following problems occur, without the important limitations noted in the "poor" category below: Generally comparable groups are assembled initially but some question remains whether some (although not major) differences occurred in follow-up; measurement instruments are acceptable (although not the best) and generally applied equally; some but not all important outcomes are considered; and some but not all potential confounders are accounted for.

Poor: Studies will be graded "poor" if any of the following major limitations exists: Groups assembled initially are not close to being comparable or maintained throughout the study; unreliable or invalid measurement instruments are used or not applied at all equally among groups (including not masking outcome assessment); and key confounders are given little or no attention.

Reviewer	Comment	Response
Question 1. Are the objectives, scope, and methods for this review clearly described?		
Bair	yes	Noted
Buffum	Overall, this synthesis is very well-written and comprehensively addresses the clearly stated key questions. The scope is slightly confusing because content from two citations contradict the exclusion criteria. Methods are clear. Exclusions: • Battlefield/emergent assessment and care (regional anesthesia being studied by Gallagher #120 covers battlefield.) Rehabilitation needs to be defined in terms of time frame or activities. • Post-traumatic/post-concussive headache unrelated to blast injury unless the sample includes patients with moderate or greater cognitive deficit. (Lew #59 reviews 5 studies about TBI but not related to blast, and cognitive impairment is not mentioned in the review. Pg 16 line 28)	We have clarified that we excluded studies describing outcomes only within 3 months of injury. Studies examining longer term outcomes of non-specific surgical treatments were included. We agree that the Lew study does not meet criteria for inclusion with main findings because it does not include studies specifically including patients with blast-related headache (or according to severity of TBI.
Clark	yes	Noted
Sayer	Objectives very clear. You may want to consider dividing KQ1 into part A and B.	Noted
Sayer	Scope/Methods: There is lack of clarity with regard to scope and methods due to the heterogeneity of polytrauma both in terms of injury constellations and injury etiology and presentation of methods and findings with regard to the composition of the samples included in the research reviewed. Below I list some specific areas where further clarification with regard to sample composition (e.g., "Polytrauma") would be helpful: see items a- f below	Noted

APPENDIX D. Reviewer comments and responses on the draft VA-ESP report on pain in polytrauma

Reviewer	Comment	Response
Sayer	a) There appears to have been inconsistency between stated study inclusion criteria (articles/research focused on pain resulting from polytraumatic injuries) and articles that were reviewed (e.g., TBI, causalgia, amputation without other injuries, blast-related headache without Polytrauma, orthopedic injuries, patients with "major trauma"). The phrase "polyrauma including TBI" is confusing to me. Do you mean that TBI = Polytrauma or that the patients had TBI that occurred in the context of other injuries. Similarly, not clear to me whether causalgia is classified as Polytrauma or whether patients with causalgia had other injuries. Does traumatic amputation = Polytrauma for the purpose of this review?	TBI of moderate to severe severity was considered polytrauma for this review, the rationale being that patients suffer from the traumatic injury itself as well as associated cognitive sequellae. Causalgia in and of itself does not meet criteria for polytrauma but as the cases included in the systematic study predominantly suffered from war-related injuries, we had included this study. However, upon further review, we feel that there is insufficient documentation in this review to consider it among the main findings, and include the results with secondary findings. Patients with unilateral injuries without evidence of other injuries were not considered to have polytrauma. Bilateral amputation was considered polytrauma in our review.
Sayer	b) Not clear on p.3 why excluding burn injuries from review. Also seems that you include burn injury in review of active research (LOBO). This is probably just a matter of clarification.	Our statement about excluding burn injuries led to confusion (and was actually not necessary). The exclusion of studies of perioperative care and surgical care encompasses the exclusion of acute treatment of burn injuries. We did not exclude studies of burn patients that examined pain related outcomes beyond perioperative care/acute burn management. We have amended the methods section accordingly.
Sayer	c) not clear to this reviewer that articles in Table 1 included patients with Polytrauma according to VA definition	TBI of moderate to severe severity is defined as polytrauma for this review. These cases studies involved patients with moderate to severe TBI or TBI concurrent with another injury/condition. Because they are case studies, these are considered secondary findings. the Table title has been changed and a footnote has been added to clarify the above.

Reviewer	Comment	Response
Sayer	d) I strongly suggest being specific with regard to sample type rather than using the general terms like "patients" or "Polytrauma patients" when summarizing findings. Given the heterogeneity of Polytrauma the term loses its usefulness for literature review purposes. For example, the summary statement on p22 would be much clearer and useful if you were specific as to sample composition.	Due to the heterogeneity of the study samples, it would be challenging to describe details of each of the included studies. However, throughout the text, we have expanded brief descriptions of samples.
Sayer	There is also some lack of clarity with regard to definition of pain related outcomes (KQ4). I do not understand reason for inclusion of psychosocial factors p 22 in context of this reviews. This is probably just a matter of clarification.	The sponsors of this review and expert panel were interested in relationships between psychosocial factors and pain-related outcomes pain intensity and pain-related disability or interference. In this review, psychosocial factors generally constitute the independent variables, and pain-related outcomes, the dependent variables. We have rewritten these sections to make this clearer.
Sayer	Other areas needing clarification and/or suggestions: a) I think you need a definition of Polytrauma that is true to your methods in the Executive Summary.	We have clarified that in addition to our main findings regarding studies that include patients meeting polytrauma criteria, we also included additional, secondary findings that may have relevance for readers of the report.
Sayer	b) I would suggest renaming Table 1 so that it is clear that it presents studies relevant to secondary findings.	See comment above. We have relabeled Table 1.
Sayer	c) I found summary of secondary findings for KQ4 confusing. I am not sure what is meant by "severity of TBI and prevalence of pain". Do you mean "presence of pain"? I was also confused by summary statement (p.18) which focuses on mild TBI. Perhaps the focus in on association between mild TBI and pain?	We have clarified that studies focusing only on mild TBI are not included in this review. We prefer the term "prevalence" to indicate the frequency of an outcome at a given point in time; some authors of included studies use the term presence instead, which in most cases, appears to indicate the same construct. We have removed the term presence when possible.
Sayer	d) not clear why you are grading the qualitative study (p.24) given your grading criteria (p.6).	The qualitative study is not given a formal grade. It is the body of evidence for Key Question 5 that was given a formal grade. We now believe that based on only one qualitative study, we should not assign a grade for the body of evidence supporting this Key Question.

Reviewer	Comment	Response
Sayer	e) I suggest adding a reference following the statement "pain is an almost universal component of polytrauma...	We have revised this section, and it no longer contains the statement cited.
Sayer	f) I am not sure of your use of the term "emergent". Perhaps OK, but I suggest confirming with trauma experts.	We have replaced the term emergent with the term "emergency". We excluded studies that only measure outcomes less than 3 months after injuries.
Schreiber	yes. 3156 citations were initially identified for review and 482 articles were retrieved. Although the authors have stated their criteria for retrieving articles, it would be helpful if they cited the reasons for excluding articles specifically. For instance, how many articles were excluded because they didn't address polytrauma patients. Similarly 482 articles were retrieved but 102 articles were included. Once again, it would be helpful if the authors specified the reasons for exclusion. For instance, how many articles were excluded because the full text could not be obtained or because the article was written in a foreign language?	We have updated the literature flow diagram in the report to contain more detail on the number of excluded articles and the reasons for exclusion.
Walker, RL	Yes, although as is described by the review committee, there was a significant challenge in finding good quality research regarding this topic in the literature.	Noted
Kerns	Yes. Although I am impressed with the effort to identify "active research" projects, I wonder if there is a potential for bias in any of several directions related to this search. For example, how extensive was the effort to identify investigators who might either be conducting relevant research involving or know of someone who is? Is there a potential bias in terms of identifying research involving persons representing certain disciplines (i.e., psychologists, primary care providers) relative to others (nurses, anesthesiologists, epidemiologists)? Was an active decision made not to make an effort to identify NIH, DoD, research foundation, or industry funded projects? Could a broader search still be accomplished, and if so, could it lead to identification of completed, but not reported, data and/or other ongoing active projects?	This is an important concern, and is addressed in a separate active research limitations section. We did attempt to identify relevant DOD studies, sending email inquires to a number of non-VA, including DOD, investigators. We additionally searched several VA and non-VA website databases: (National Institutes of Health Clinical Trials data base (http:www.clinicaltrials.gov), the Computer Retrieval of Information on Scientific Projects (CRISP) database, Current Controlled Trials (http://www.controlled-trials.com/mrct/), and the VA HSR&D website (http://www.hsrd.research.va.gov/research/default.c fm). We have included more informationo about our search strategies and email contacts in the report.

Question 2. Is there any indication of bias in our synthesis of the evidence?

Reviewer	Comment	Response
Bair	no	Noted
Buffum	Probably not bias: Question 1 needs some clarity in defining cognitive impairment. Cognitive impairment early in rehab is not differentiated from acute...the emphasis seems to be more on chronic but it is not differentiated. Also, cognitive impairment in dementia needs more distinction for pain reporting. (pg 11 lines 3-4). Is there an MMSE cutoff where patients cannot self-report reliably? (this differs by author and is biased for language and education so doesn't apply to everyone) If dementia is categorized as mild or moderate, that might help....most patients within these categories can understand (but not all).	Detailed exploration of these complex issues is beyond the scope of this review, especially as this section presents secondary findings from the review. We have shortened this section. We have clarified some of the statements with regard to patients having mild to severe levels of dementia.
Buffum	Pg 11 lines 14-20: there are actually 4 reviews now (2 international—Zwakhalen et al, 2006 and vanHerk et al, 2007) and (2 U.S.—Herr et al, 2006 and Stolee et al, 2005). Stolee, Herr, and vanHerk state the Discomfort Scale is most psychometrically sound (and Herr adds NOPPAIN). Zwakhalen and vanHerk refer to the PACSLAC as being best. Only van Herk says PAINAD is promising, and Herr says this about PACSLAC. So, it might be fair to say that there are U.S. and international differences. And the synthesis is correct that there is no one best tool! Additionally, it might be beneficial to state that multiple methods are best for assessment....which address all of the items mentioned in lines 17-20. Cohen-Mansfield's 2008 article addresses the notion that multiple methods may be better than any single tool. Reviews of tools concur that most are tested in few studies, studies are small, not all patients have all behaviors, and new tools tend to be developed before old ones are tested. Newer tools seem to address better pain intensity, function, activity when pain behaviors are noted, and effect of specific intervention.	We have updated this section. We have reviewed the suggested manuscripts and incorporated their findings. See response above for more information.
Buffum	Also, it might be helpful to indicate that the tools for geriatrics (dementia) are rated on how well they adhere to the American Geriatrics Society Guidelines. Similar guidelines are not available specifically for TBI but other populations and issues are addressed in the ASPMN statement: Herr K. Pain assessment in the nonverbal patient: position statement with clinical practice recommendations. Pain Manage Nurs. 2006;7(2):44-52.	See above two responses.
Clark	Not bias, but some misleading statements or conclusions: a. P. 12, lines 18-20, as well as this entire section, does not address the issue of the transient effects of these treatments. In fact, the "94%...were cured" statement, which I'm sure comes from the article itself, is highly, highly unlikely since even a "successful" sympathectomy typically does not "cure" pain in that, on average, pain recurs within an 8 to 14 month period (there are numerous studies examining long-term effects of sympathectomies in the literature, including a recent Cochrane review). In fact, the use of this treatment for neuropathic pain is controversial. Blocks (rather than destruction) also are temporary, when they work at all, and endless repeat blocks or ESIs (a common practice) have other potential risks (see recent Neurology review and guidelines).	Due to questions about whether the studies included in this review clearly include patients with polytrauma, we now consider this study's findings to be secondary findings. We have added an additional statement noting the limitations of this study's findings.

APPENDIX D. Reviewer comments and responses on the draft VA-ESP report on pain in polytrauma

Reviewer	Comment	Response
Clark (Continued)	My point here is that I think it would be unwise to leave the reader with the impression that these procedures are all that efficacious or even, in some cases, recommended, and that effectiveness proof requires not only high quality RCTs but also temporal follow up to determine the stability of the effects.	See above response.
Clark	b. On p. 15, lines 6-32, were these patients assessed for other kinds of pain beyond headaches? The last sentence reports that PTSD and depression were identified as mediators (or should they be moderators?) of physical health problems rather than headaches in general, but does not indicate whether pain other than headache (which also is common following blast exposure) was assessed. If not, it would be hard to attribute physical health effects mostly to PTSD or depression.	This study assessed patients for a number of somatic symptoms in addition to pain. We have changed the wording regarding the findings of this study. It is not possible to say conclusively how PTSD and depression are associated with pain. We now more carefully state, "the associations among TBI and physical health problems are no longer significant when PTSD and depression are included in models."
Sayer	It is difficult to evaluate the active research for the obvious reason that there are no publications or other products other than the objectives of the study, which are always lofty. The review of active research may give the impression that all gaps will be filled in the near future. I am not sure of that. In many of these studies pain is a secondary outcome and the quality of pain data will be limited. I suggest that you include in Table 2 an indicator of whether the pain outcome is primary/secondary and in your review that you discuss potential limitations associated with many of these active studies (particularly in the limitation section). For example, at least one of the studies is a QI project (Kerns PI) This study will help improve practice, I believe, but I am not sure that it will address KQ1&5 in a generalizeable way. I also think it may be helpful to have the grant #s listed in the reference section as there may be some errors.	We have added a column to Table 2 indicating whether pain-related outcomes are a primary or secondary focus of each study. We will also address these important concerns in a separate limitations section included within the active research section. We will include grant numbers and agencies when available.
Schreiber	No, The review is extremely comprehensive with broad representation of literature from all sectors. There is no evidence of bias.	Noted
Walker, RL	No, the reviewers appeared to provide a balanced review of the evidence that is available at this time.	Noted
Kerns	No; except with regard to the identification of active research projects as described above.	Noted
Question 3. Are there any studies on pain in patients with polytrauma that we have overlooked?		
Bair	not, that I know about	Noted
Buffum	Not that I know of. Very comprehensively addressed.	Noted
Clark	None that I know of.	Noted

Reviewer	Comment	Response
Schreiber	There is a prospective cohort study on outcome after amputation: Bosse et al, NEJM. 2002;347:1924-1931. This article may have been excluded because it does not mention polytrauma or because it focuses on surgical technique. However, this article is prospective and it give 2 year outcome data in a large amputation population (569 patients). Failure to include articles like this would seem to be a weakness of this review.	We reviewed the suggested study at the full-text level and were not able to include it in our review because pain was not an outcome.
Walker, RL	Not that I am aware of in the current published or non-published literature	Noted
Kerns	None of which I am aware	Noted
Question 4. Future research recommendations table, by key question		
KQ1. Are pain assessment tools reliable and valid in patients with cognitive deficits due to TBI?		
Buffum	Partnership with family to identify pain behaviors and responses rial of protocol specific to identified pain behaviors such as that used in dementia (Serial Trials Intevention--Kovach et al)--- Include in a tool items found helpful in dementia: combinations (observation, self-report, family report, combination, empiric analgesic, all of these; function, intensity, triggering situations, co-morbidities –both physical and psychological) Qualitative study to identify pain behaviors in different cognitively impaired TBI states. Develop a new tool (match severity and type of cognitive impairment) Evaluate use of the dementia tools in TBI What other tools provide some utility?(unconscious patients in ICU?infants?)	Noted, and included
Clark	Highly needed, but all research in this area suffers from the same problem: What do you use as a criterion when assessing measure validity when patients cannot provide self-reports? Observational studies are the hallmark but generally cannot distinguish between pain-related or dementia/TBI-related behaviors such as agitation, restlessness, etc	Noted
Sayer	Table 4. Why are you recommending qualitative studies to address KQ1?	Qualitative studies often generate hypotheses for subsequent quantitative testing. For example as noted by another reviewer, a qualitative study for Key Question 1 examining pain behaviors/responses identified by family members might lead to development of a new tool for assessing pain in TBI patients.

APPENDIX D. Reviewer comments and responses on the draft VA-ESP report on pain in polytrauma

Reviewer	Comment	Response
Schreiber	Develop an assessment tool that differentiates symptoms of TBI from PTSD. Some degree of TBI screening is being performed on injured soldiers being admitted to Landstuhl Regional Medical Center	Noted. We are focusing in this set of research recommendations on evaluation of measures for pain. We will include a research topic on assessing discriminant validity of pain assessment tools.
Kerns	Studies of pain assessment during coma emergence may be an interesting paradigm in which to study the reliability and validity of these assessment tools. Examination of moderators of reliability of the tools including examination of TBI/cognitive dysfunction severity should be encouraged. A key question is the discriminant validity of these assessment tools for distinguishing pain and forms of emotional distress. This should be explicitly stated as an important area for research. A specific strategy for assessment of the validity of these tools is to employ them in the context of clinical trials of pain interventions. That is, evidence for the validity of the measure can come from evidence of declining "pain ratings" in conjunction with delivery of opioid analgesics, for example. As a follow-up to the qualitative study in the PRCs, explicit examination of the reliability, validity, and utility of the module for the assessment of pain among non-communicative patients is indicated.	Noted and included

KQ2a. Which treatments improve pain outcomes in polytrauma patients?

Reviewer	Comment	Response
Clark	Trials of telephone-based interventions?	Noted and included
Kerns	Of particular relevance are studies of opioids, since these medications are likely to be used with considerable frequency, are presumed to be associated with increased cognitive dysfunction that may undermine rehabilitation efforts, and are associated with safety risks including respiratory depression, abuse and addiction, and diversion. However, studies of the efficacy of nonpharmacological interventions, especially psychological interventions, are indicated. It seems that virtually any prospective randomized controlled trial in this area is indicated. Systematic prospective observational studies and single case experimental designs with replication may be more likely given the heterogeneity of the population and the relatively small numbers of persons who could be enrolled at one or even a few sites.	Noted and included

KQ2b. Which pain treatment approaches enhance overall rehabilitation efforts?

APPENDIX D. Reviewer comments and responses on the draft VA-ESP report on pain in polytrauma

Reviewer	Comment	Response
Clark	RCTs examining a range of treatment approaches including comprehensive interdisciplinary rehab. Additionally, comparisons of Tx for specific conditions (e.g., TBI; PTSD; Pain) could be compared to more general treatment of the core of overlapping symptoms that characterize this polytrauma triad of symptoms (e.g., the "P3" Tx model developed at Tampa). Comparisons of standard vs. low Tx intensity impact.	Noted and included
Kerns	The relationship between improved pain control and rehabilitation outcomes is an important target. Again, systematic prospective observation methods and single case experimental designs with replication are likely to be most useful in this regard.	Noted and included
KQ3a. Does blast-related headache pain differ from other types of headache pain?		
Buffum	Impact of comorbid psych issues on headache in these patients (e.g., PTSD or schizophrenia with auditory hallucinations)---	Noted and included
Clark	Obviously, prospective studies are difficult here unless one follows a large number of deployed soldiers pre and post. More practical would be comparisons of Sx between those with "migraine-like" or "tension-like" post-traumatic headaches and non-posttraumatic migraine and tension HAs, or between those with blast and non-blast post-traumatic HAs	Noted and included
Schreiber	Perform routine imaging on soldiers exposed to blast to assess for structural abnormalities and correlate with headache symptoms	Noted and included
Kerns	A carefully designed cross-sectional study of veterans with either headache presumed to be related to blast-injury or with headache not known to be associated with blast would likely be important and have a high impact.	Noted and included
KQ3b. Which treatments are best for persistent blast-related headache pain?		
Clark	Typical HA meds do not seem to be as effective with this cohort according to treating clinicians. Therefore, trials of new meds (or new applications of meds), as well as additive or subtractive studies of meds +- CBT would be useful.	Noted and included
Schreiber	Prospective randomized trials using different pain strategies in patients with blast-related headache pain	Noted and included
Kerns	An RCT of psychological interventions for blast-related headache is feasible and strongly indicated given evidence for the efficacy of similar interventions in other headache populations. Interventions including hypnosis, relaxation training, biofeedback, and cognitive-behavior therapy are particularly indicated.	Noted and included
KQ4a. What patient factors are associated with better and worse (pain-related) clinical outcomes among polytrauma patients?		

APPENDIX D. Reviewer comments and responses on the draft VA-ESP report on pain in polytrauma

Reviewer	Comment	Response
Clark	1. Validate value of typical pain outcomes predictors (e.g., depression; catastrophizing; fear; etc.) in this cohort. 2. Comparisons of pain course between polytrauma and non-polytrauma patients matched by pain type/location 3. Associations between pain and PTSD and pain and TBI.	Noted and included
Buffum	Partnership with family?	Noted and included
Schreiber	Develop a comprehensive survey tool given to soldiers prior to deployment that includes questions concerning prior injuries, history of pain related issues, medication history, etc. Couple this with the post-deployment assessments at the time of re-deployment and 6 months later.	Noted and included
KQ4b. Have interventions been developed to specifically address these factors?		
Clark	Identify factors first.	Noted and included
Kerns	An RCT of psychological interventions for blast-related headache is feasible and strongly indicated given evidence for the efficacy of similar interventions in other headache populations. Interventions including hypnosis, relaxation training, biofeedback, and cognitive-behavior therapy are particularly indicated.	Noted and included
KQ5a. What are unique provider and system barriers to detecting and treating pain among polytrauma patients? Have interventions been developed to effectively address these barriers?		
Buffum	What is the role for nonpharmacologic measures? (hypnosis, acupuncture, massage, music, exercise)---- What cultural adaptations(or acceptance of diversity) are the PRCs doing to accomodate patients with pain? (e.g. cultural or religious practices)	Noted and included
Clark	1. Impact of polytrauma pain education on provider behavior. 2. Establishment and subsequent testing of expert opinion Tx guidelines. 3. Evaluations of patient perceived barriers and impact of efforts to mitigate those barriers.	Noted and included
Kerns	Follow-up of the qualitative study in the PRCs will be important to further examine implementation of CPRS tools for pain assessment. A specific focus on overcoming physician barriers to the conduct of pain assessments in this, and other populations, will be important. Further refinement of the tools to improve provider/nursing use and satisfaction with the tools is likely indicated	Noted and included
Sayer	For KQ5 I suggest organizational research.	Noted and included
Question 5a (review form). Additional Suggestions for future research		

APPENDIX D. Reviewer comments and responses on the draft VA-ESP report on pain in polytrauma

Reviewer	Comment	Response
Bair	Informed by this excellent review, I think it would be helpful to hold a consensus meeting(s) based on the IMMPACT group (Initiative on Methods, Measurement, and Pain Assessment in Clinical Trials) to develop consensus recommendations and priorities to populate the table and provide future research recommendations.	We compiled a list of reviewers' recommendations for specific studies, and sent this list to the expert panel to help prioritize. Because these are preliminary rankings, a panel or other mechanism to achieve consensus is needed to refine and finalize the recommendations for future research.
Buffum	My suggestions are in double columns for Question 1. Wherever partnership with family could be studied as an intervention, I'd suggest that for future research. The role of distraction, nonpharmacologic methods, elements of rehab that are most successful for these pts with multiple injuries including neurological and psychological trauma	Noted and included
Clark	As we knew from the outset, there is little direct research in the general area of polytrauma pain despite the fact that multiple traumas of one type or another have occurred for centuries. Typically trauma medicine is more concerned with survival than pain, rightly so to a degree. But acute-phase pain interventions may offer the most long term benefit for patients in terms of prevention of chronic pain or minimization of its associated disabilities. So one area of valuable research clearly involves this relatively unknown acute phase. Mac's study tries to address this from one perspective, but a variety of other areas are ripe for exploration as well (eventual impact of improved pain care on or near the battlefield; associations between acute injury pain and injury related emotional issues; etc.). (CONTINUED NEXT ROW)	Noted and included. We have added additional statements regarding the advisability of improving VA-DoD collaborations in our research recommendations section.
Clark (Continued)	The challenge is that almost all of these studies would need to involve BOTH the DoD and VA, and despite occasional reports to the contrary, we have far from a close working relationship between the two. So another priority for me would be to try to foster DoD/VA linkage in the area of pain care similar to initial linkages that have been made in other OEF/OIF care issues (e.g., ID; vascular; surgery; psychiatry). Though not related specifically to research, perhaps a joint DoD/VA working conference or joint work group focusing on identifying ways to collaborate more effectively in pain research would be helpful. Right now, some of us attend some of the annual military medical conferences, but pain rarely is attended to in any detail. Just a thought.	See above.

Reviewer	Comment	Response
Schreiber	1. There is an enormous amount of information that is already available that could be mined for future research. All soldiers returning from deployment undergo a post-deployment assessment questionnaire just prior to leaving the field and 6 months later. Although, the questions are limited, they may provide important insight into later outcomes. These questionnaires could also be modified to make them more useful. 2. Most soldiers undergo pre and post-deployment hearing tests. Soldiers who are not exposed to blast injury could serve as controls for those who are to determine if all of the hearing loss is related to blast injury. For example, my hearing worsened after my deployment and I was not exposed to blast injury. (CONTINUED NEXT ROW)	We have incorporated these ideas into our research recommendation section.
Schreiber (continued)	Additional screening should be routinely performed on soldiers admitted to Landstuhl Regional Medical Center. All injured soldiers from Iraq and Afghanistan go through LRMC and as a Level 4 facility this is a tremendous opportunity to collect data. 4. It is my understanding that all deploying soldiers have a blood sample taken and stored prior to deployment. This provides an incredible opportunity to study genetic factors associated with chronic pain, PTSD and outcome after TBI. This could result in opportunities for intervention	See above.

Question 5b (review form). Additional comments

Bair	Thank you for highlighting our ESCAPE study in the review. The only suggestion that I have is to include that the comparator is "treatment as usual" or "usual care." 1. Page V (executive summary), Line 37: Suggest adding "ICU" to length of stay to improve clarity	Correction made. Correction made.
Bair	2. Page 1, Line 45: Minor typo. Suggest changing first word from On to Among	Correction made.
Bair	3. Page 2, Line 23: add undiscovered shrapnel fragments	Correction made.
Bair	4. Page 4—I like the analytic framework diagram. Suggest a minor edit to include a legend noting that KQ = Key Question	Correction made.
Bair	5. Page 7: Capitalize GRADE (The Grading of Recommendations, Assessment, Development, and Evaluation (GRADE) Working Group—suggest also to write out the acronym	Correction made.
Bair	6. Page 9—I like the diagram, but a one-word descriptor of each KQ may help the reader. For example under KQ1 you might include Assessment	Correction made.

APPENDIX D. Reviewer comments and responses on the draft VA-ESP report on pain in polytrauma

Reviewer	Comment	Response
Bair	7. Page 12 (lines 28 to 32). Why was no p-value reported for the greater HRQL outcome? In addition, I think the remaining discussion is slightly misleading. The p-values for "increased likelihood to return to work" and "reduced hours of work" were not statistically significant. It may be more accurate to say there was a "trend" towards statistical significance for these outcomes. This should also be changed in the conclusion table.	We have revised the sentence to read as follows: After controlling for demographic factors, injury characteristics and other medical morbidity, inpatient rehabilitation was marginally associated with increased likelihood of return to work (p=0.09) and decreased likelihood of reduced hours of work (p=0.05).
Bair	8. Pages 13 and 14, Table 1: Is the outcome "global improvement" a patient self-reported or clinician reported outcome?	We have confirmed the global improvement outcome was clinician-reported in this study and have indicated this on Table 1.
Bair	9. Page 14, Lines 39 and 40: There is some redundancy here (e.g. "in the review" is mentioned twice).	Correction made.
Bair	10. Page 17, Line 24: Add "ICU" length of stay	Correction made.
Bair	11. Style point: I might consider more liberal use of bulleted text, especially when describing several studies	Noted.
Bair	12. Page 21, Lines 28 to 30: Not sure how to edit, but the current wording is awkward	Correction made.
Bair	13. Page 21, Lines 32 to 34: Suggest edit to say something like "multiply and singly injured patients to reduce redundancy	Correction made.
Bair	14. Page 23, Line 31: Edit percentages reported—e.g., 44% to 54% and (line 34) 17% to 18%	Correction made.
Bair	15. Page 23, Line 41: Pain scores are reported but not sure what is the range of scores here? 0 to 100 scale?	The suggested has been added.
Bair	16. Page 23, line 42: Suggest using the term prevalence instead of "frequency."	Correction made.
Bair	17. Page 32, table 3: I like the summary table. It is clear and concise. However, the results of 2b are not all statistically significant and thus may be misleading	We have changed the wording in Table 3 to be more consistent with the findings.

APPENDIX D. Reviewer comments and responses on the draft VA-ESP report on pain in polytrauma

Reviewer	Comment	Response
Buffum	Here are some details I noticed as I read: Pg iv line 4 this appears to contradict pg 5 line 46 ?	Pg iv line 4: We systematically rated the quality of cohort and case-control design studies. pg 5 lines 43-46: Due to a limited number of studies that included a comparator group, we also considered relevant cross-sectional and case report/case series studies for inclusion for some of the key questions. For these study designs, data were not formally abstracted nor rated for quality of evidence. Response: The former sentence refers to case-control studies which include a comparator group, whereas the latter refers to case reports/case series that do not include a comparator group.
Buffum	Pg 12 line 30 p value for QOL?	The result has been clarified.
Buffum	Pg 12 #36 and #52 what is complex regional pain syndrome 1? In text it is always 2.	Complex Regional Pain Syndrome 1 is the syndrome previously known as regional sympathetic dystrophy. Complex Regional Pain Syndrome was previously known as causalgia. We have referred to these older labels when first introducing these syndromes.
Buffum	Pg 19 line 22 headache "density" (should it be "intensity"?) Lines 30-34 inconsistency of p value and r.	Density is the term used by the study author (Walker 2005). We have defined his usage of the density in the text. The p-value in line 31 and the r-value in line 35 refer to the results of separate studies.
Buffum	Pg 22 line 30 to summarize, there "are" …. (should it be "is"?)	Correction made.
Buffum	Pg 26 2nd to last row on the bottom (127) in 2nd column: Compare cost costs. (delete "cost")	Correction made.
Buffum	Pg 31 line 7 Two librarians independently search…. (should be "searched"?)	Correction made.
Buffum	Pg 32 Key Question 1 second bullet….Most patients with mild cognitive impairment … (add "mild") Add a bullet: There is no evidence that pain assessment tools for dementia could be reliably applied to persons with cognitive impairment related to TBI.	Correction made.

10/5/2010

APPENDIX D. Reviewer comments and responses on the draft VA-ESP report on pain in polytrauma

Reviewer	Comment	Response
Helmer	I was a little taken aback by your summary of the Hoge TBI paper (ref 54) on page 15. "overall, the analyses suggest that...high rates of physical health problems...are mediated largely by PTSD and depression." "Mediated" doesn't necessarily imply causality, of course, but I think you need to be a little more careful about stating it in such a way to not be interpreted as "PTSD and depression explain the high rates of physical health problems." How about the associations between TBI and physical health problems were no longer significant after inclusion of PTSD and depression?	We agree and have corrected the error.

Reviewers

Bair	Matthew J. Bair, MD, MS
Buffum	Martha Buffum, DNSC, APRN, BC, CS
Clark	Michael E. Clark, Ph.D.
Helmer	Drew Helmer, M.D.
Kerns	Robert Kerns, Ph.D.
Otis	John D. Otis, Ph.D.
Sayer	Nina Sayer, Ph.D.
Schreiber	Martin A. Schreiber, MD
Walker, RL	Robyn L. Walker, Ph.D.

APPENDIX E, EVIDENCE TABLE 1. Studies on patient factors associated with polytrauma outcomes (Key Question 4)

Author, Year (ref.)	Title	Topic area	Study Design	Sample: All polytrauma patients, majority, or just included?	Aims
TBI					
Bay, 2008(1)	Risk factors for depressive symptoms after mild-to-moderate traumatic brain injury	TBI	Cross sectional	Included	To determine the extent to which pre-injury psychosocial factors, injury-related variables and post-injury litigation, perceived stress, fatigue, pain and information processing speed contributed to depressive symptoms after traumatic brain injury(TBI)
Beetar, 1996(2)	Sleep and Pain Complaints in Symptomatic Traumatic Brain Injury and Neurological Populations	TBI, fatigue, insomnia	Case-contol	Included	To compare the incidence of sleep and pain complaints in symptomatic taumatic brain injury(TBI) (mils vs. moderate/severe) and neurologic populations
Brenner, 1944(3)	Post-traumatic Headache	TBI, headache	Cohort--prospective	Majority	Study relationships among manner and degree of head injury, personality factors, compensation, environmental status and headache prevalence and course.
Bryant, 1999(4)	Interaction of Posttraumatic Stress Disorder and Chronic Pain following Traumatic Brain Injury	TBI, PSTD	Cohort--prospective	All (severe TBI)	To investigate the association between PTSD and chronic pain in patients who had sustained a severe TBI
Bushnik, 2008(5)	The Experience of Fatigue in the First 2 years After Moderate-to-Severe traumatic Brain Injury: A Preliminary Report	TBI, fatigue/ insomnia	Cohort--prospective	All	This study examined the rate and tyes of fatigue that are experienced by a cohort of individuals w. TBI within the first 2 years using a multidimensional fatigue scale. The impact of factors such as demographics, injury severity indices and concomtant psychosocial variables was also examined.

APPENDIX E, EVIDENCE TABLE 1. Stud es on patient factors associated with polytrauma outcomes (Key Question 4)

Author, Year (ref.)	Setting	Sample demographics and other characteristics (include average time since injury at study baseline, if applicable)	Inclusion/exclusion criteria
TBI			
Bay, 2008(1)	8 outpatient rehabilitation cneters in the Midwest	49% female, 89% white, 77% Glascow Coma Scale (GCS) score 13-15, 45% with CT findings, average 15 months since injury, ave age=38	Inclusion: 1-36 months from date of injury;hospitalized or seen in ER at time of injury Exclusion: preexisting neurologic /cognitive disorders; severe TBI
Beetar, 1996(2)	Outpatient neuropsychological service at a university affiliated tertiary care center	TBI group: age 36, 68 % male , 24 months post-injury	Cases: patients consectively referred for neuropsychological assessment w. TBI, Controls: referred pts without TBI
Brenner, 1944(3)	Boston City Hospital	63% males, 36% Irish, 48% skilled or semi-skilled workers	Inclusion: 200 consecutive patients with head injury admitted to hospital, age 15 to 55. Exclude: unemployed and with chronic alcoholism
Bryant, 1999(4)	Tertiary Care Center, Brain Injury Clinic	80% male, age not specified	Inclusion: admitted to brain injury rehab with severe TBI
Bushnik, 2008(5)	TBI inpatient rehabilitation service	74% male, age 34	Inclusion: TBI, admitted to inpatient rehab., Exclusion: medical disorders associated with fatigue

APPENDIX E, EVIDENCE TABLE 1. Studies on patient factors associated with polytrauma outcomes (Key Question 4)

Author, Year (ref.)	N enrolled, Tx v. controls	Exposure of interest	Control group: Comparator to exposure of interest	Pain-related outcomes measured	Timing of Outcomes	Is pain outcome a **main** outcome in
TBI						
Bay, 2008(1)	84	n/a	n/a	McGill Pain Questionaire short form	Single assessment Ave. 15 months post-injury	No
Beetar, 1996(2)	202 TBI pts and 123 non-TBI pts.	non-TBI TBI	non-TBI	prevalence of pain complaints	Single assessment, av e. 24 months post-injury	No
Brenner, 1944(3)	200 enrolled	n/a	none	headache prevalence	During admission, before 2 months, then every 2 months up to 6 to 15 months	Yes
Bryant, 1999(4)	96	PTSD with TBI	non PTSD with TBI	10 pt VAS-pain intensity, location, frequency	6 months	Yes
Bushnik, 2008(5)	38	n/a	n/a	VAS 10 pt. Scale	1 & 2 yrs.	No

APPENDIX E, EVIDENCE TABLE 1. Studies on patient factors associated with polytrauma outcomes (Key Question 4)

Author, Year (ref.)	Are results stratified or adjusted for polytrauma	Analytic method	Variables adjusted for in analysis or stratification
TBI			
Bay, 2008(1)	No	multiple regression techniques	Perceived stress, impact of events, litigation status
Beetar, 1996(2)	by TBI severity	bivariate tests	TBI severity
Brenner, 1944(3)	n/a--majority with polytrauma	descriptive only	Head injury severity as measured by duration of post-traumatic amnesia, coma, and disorientation
Bryant, 1999(4)	All polytrauma patients	partial correlation coefficients and chi square	PSTD
Bushnik, 2008(5)	All polytrauma patients	bivariate	None

APPENDIX E, EVIDENCE TABLE 1. Studies on patient factors associated with polytrauma outcomes (Key Question 4)

Author, Year (ref.)	Results	Quality rating
TBI		
Bay, 2008(1)	In a model including perceived stress, impact of events, and litigation stress, pain was significantly associated with depression(partial R(squared)=.07, p=.001)	n/a--cross-sectional
Beetar, 1996(2)	TBI subjects had significantly more insomnia (56.4% vs. 30.9%) and pain complaints (58.9% vs. 22%) than non-TBI subjects(p< .0001). For both subject groups, the presence of pain increased insomnia approximately twofold.	Fair
Brenner, 1944(3)	69% of patients reported headaches while in hospital and 41% reported headaches after hospitalization. There was no greater prevalence of headache persisting longer than two months among patients with more severe head injuries than patients with milder head injuries.	Fair
Bryant, 1999(4)	More patients who reported chronic pain (37%) met criteria for PTSD than did those without pain (15%), chi-squre=5.70, p<.05. Frequency but not severity of chronic pain was associated with PTSD (p<.05)	Fair
Bushnik, 2008(5)	There were highly significant correlations between levels of fatigue and pain at one and 2 years post-injury (R=.49 and .62, respectively, p<.01)	Poor

APPENDIX E, EVIDENCE TABLE 1. Studies on patient factors associated with polytrauma outcomes (Key Question 4)

Author, Year (ref.)	Title	Topic area	Study Design	Sample: All polytrauma patients, majority, or just included?	Aims
Cantor, 2008(6)	Fatigue After Traumatic Brain Injury and Its Impact on Participation and Quality of Life	TBI, fatigue	Case-control	Included (mild to severe TBI)	To examine the relationships between post-TBI fatigue and comorbid conditions, participation in activities, quality of life, and demographic and injury variables
Cosgrove, 1989(7)	A Prospective study of Peripheral Nerve Lesions occurring in Traumatic Brain-injured Patients	causalgia, complex regional/causalgia /autonom, TBI	Cohort-prospective	All	The purpose of this study was to determine the frequency and severity of peripheral nerve lesions occurring in pateint withtraumatic brain injury.
Dawson, 2007(8)	Return to productivity following traumatic brain injury: Cognitive, psychological, physical spiritual, and environmental correlates	TBI	Cohort--prospective	Included (about 1/2 with > mild TBI)	The purpose of this study was to investigate the determinants and correlates of return to productivity (RTP) defined here as return to paid employment and/or school four years following traumatic brain injury(TBI)
Guttman, 1943(9)	Postconcussional Headache	TBI, headache	Cohort--retrospective	Included: mild to severe TBI	Describe prevalence of headaches in patient with head injury over time
Hillier, 1997(10)	Outcomes 5 years post-traumatic brain injury (with further reference to neurophysical impairment and disability)	TBI, headache	Cohort -- retrospective	Included: mild to severe TBI	This study collected data on people who had sustained a TBI 5 yrs. previously. Broad outcomes were investigated as well as the specific nature and prevalence of any residual physical impairment and disability

APPENDIX E, EVIDENCE TABLE 1. Studies on patient factors associated with polytrauma outcomes (Key Question 4)

Author, Year (ref.)	Setting	Sample demographics and other characteristics (include average time since injury at study baseline, if applicable)	Inclusion/exclusion criteria
Cantor, 2008(6)	community sample recruited with flyers and advertisements from brain injury clinic	Cases: 53% male , 41% AA, 40% white, 62% severe TBI, age 47.8 Controls: 70% male, 33% AA, 40% white, age 43.0	Case: Include--TBI, >= 12 months postinjury ,Exclude: history of non-traumatic brain injury Controls: no history of brain injury
Cosgrove, 1989(7)	single site inpatient TBI rehabilitaion center	none reported	consecutive pts. admitted to the center
Dawson, 2007(8)	Large regional trauma center	52% w. mild TBI (others w. more severe TBI), age 27.6, 54% male	Subjects enrolled consecutively over 15 months. Inclusion: non-penetrating TBI, age 16-65, responsive within 1 month of injury Exclusion: previous neurological disorder drug or alcohol abuse, history of illness
Guttman, 1943(9)	1 site-- admitted to accident service of infirmary	MVA in 77%	Inclusion: patients admitted for head injury, nonservice cases
Hillier, 1997(10)	TBI admissions to teaching hospital	age 28.9, 84% male, 69% injuries related to MVA	inclusion: TBI sustained 5 years previously

APPENDIX E, EVIDENCE TABLE 1. Studies on patient factors associated with polytrauma outcomes (Key Question 4)

Author, Year (ref.)	N enrolled, Tx v. controls	Exposure of interest	Control group: Comparator to exposure of interest	Pain-related outcomes measured	Timing of Outcomes	Is pain outcome a __main__ outcome in
Cantor, 2008(6)	223 cases, 85 controls	TBI	no TBI	McGill pain questionaire; SF 36 bodily pain	cross-sectional: average of 15 yrs. after injury	No
Cosgrove, 1989(7)	132 patients, 13 with peripheral nerve injuries	n/a	none	presence and types of pain	variable	No
Dawson, 2007(8)	94 enrolled; (47 participated , 50% flu interviews	n/a	n/a	Westhaven--Yale multidimensional pain inventory	Cross-sectional Ave. 4.3 yrs after injury	No
Guttman, 1943(9)	158	---	---	documentation of headaches	3 and 6 months after injury	Yes
Hillier, 1997(10)	67	n/a	n/a	self report prevalence of pain/location	5 years	No

10/5/2010

APPENDIX E, EVIDENCE TABLE 1. Studies on patient factors associated with polytrauma outcomes (Key Question 4)

Author, Year (ref.)	Are results stratified or adjusted for polytrauma	Analytic method	Variables adjusted for in analysis or stratification
Cantor, 2008(6)	No	correlations & multivariate regression	Overlap variables, depression sleep score, McGill pain subscales 5 fatigue items
Cosgrove, 1989(7)	No	basic descriptive, no comparisons	None
Dawson, 2007(8)	Yes	multivariate regression	Severity of TBI, time to recovery of free recall, depression, pain, coping, stroop interference time
Guttman, 1943(9)	by Head injury severity	descriptive	None
Hillier, 1997(10)	No	descriptive	None

APPENDIX E, EVIDENCE TABLE 1. Studies on patient factors associated with polytrauma outcomes (Key Question 4)

Author, Year (ref.)	Results	Quality rating
Cantor, 2008(6)	pain is associated w. TBI TBI v. Controls: adjusted McGill pain index rating 17.23 vs. 10.10 (p=.013) SF-36 health survey, bodily pain: 64.7 v. 83.2 (p<0.001) post-TBI fatigue has a signif cant impact on quality of life and well being that are not accounted for by pain, depression and sleep disturbance alone.	Fair
Cosgrove, 1989(7)	1. 13 of 132 pateints found to have peripheral nerve injuries 2. 4 of 13 pateints with peripherla nerve injuries had pain, 2 with causalgia, 2 with coplex regional pain syndrome I	Poor
Dawson, 2007(8)	Spearman's rank correlation coefficient (r) for association between pain and return to productivity: All TBI: 0.50 (p=0.0004) Mild TBI: 0.45 (p=0.03) Mod/Sev TBI: 0.65 (p=0.001) For every unit increase in the log of pain, the odds of going back to work are reduced by 96%. In post-hoc analyses, pain was highly correlated with depression (r=.081).	Fair
Guttman, 1943(9)	There was no difference in headache prevalence according to head injury severity at 6 months	Poor
Hillier, 1997(10)	58% of patients had headaches 5 years after TBI. 5% had decreased movement w. musculoskeletal pain	Poor

APPENDIX E, EVIDENCE TABLE 1. Studies on patient factors associated with polytrauma outcomes (Key Question 4)

Author, Year (ref.)	Title	Topic area	Study Design	Sample: All polytrauma patients, majority, or just included?	Aims
Hoffman, 2007(11)	Understanding Pain After Traumatic brain Injury	TBI	Cohort--prospective	Included (moderate to severe TBI)	To determine the prevalence of pain at 1 year after injury using a secondary analysis of a prospectively collected sample and to examine possible factors related to overall pain reports in individuals w. TBI. Possible predictors of pain at 1 year were examined as well as factors associated w. pain at 1 yr.. In addition, the relationship of apin, depression, and community participation was explored
Lippert-Gruner, 2007(12)	Health-related quality of life during the first year after severe brain trauma with and without polytrauma	TBI	Case control	All	Investigate health related quality of life in TBI pts with and without additional injuries
Masson, 1996(13)	Prevalence of impairments 5 years after a head injury, and their relationship with disabilities and outcome	TBI	Cohort--prospective	All	To determine what consequences cognitive behavioral or somatic complaints had on disabilities and recovery after head injury
Olver, 1996(14)	Outcome following traumatic brain injury: a comparison between 2 and 5 years after injury	TBI, headache	Cohort--retrospective	Included	This study examined longterm outcomes in traumatically brain-injured individuals following discharge from a comprehensive rehabilitation programme.
Walker, 2005(15)	Headache After Moderate and Severe Traumatic Brain Injury: A Longitudinal Analysis	TBI, headache	Cohort--prospective	All	Main objectives were to describe posttraumatic headache in acute rehabilitation patients with moderate and severe TBI and assess the course of post-traumatic headache over time.

OTHER INJURIES

APPENDIX E, EVIDENCE TABLE 1. Studies on patient factors associated with polytrauma outcomes (Key Question 4)

Author, Year (ref.)	Setting	Sample demographics and other characteristics (include average time since injury at study baseline, if applicable)	Inclusion/exclusion criteria
Hoffman, 2007(11)	single site, university brain injury program	Mean age 36.1, 76% male,78% white, mean # of injuries assoc. with TBI=2.0 23 of 202 subjects were lost to follow-up. Those who did not complete the SF-36 were more likely to be nonwhite.	Inclusion: primary diagnosis of TBI, age >16, received acute & inpatient rehab care
Lippert-Gruner, 2007(12)	Not specified	Not specified	Not specified
Masson, 1996(13)	admission to 1 of 3 trauma centers in France	51% age 15-29, 29% 30-44,19% 45-59, 75% male, 72% injured in MVA	Inclusion: patients admitted to trauma center with multiple injuries including head injury, age >15and <60
Olver, 1996(14)	Comprehensive rehabilitation programme	65% male, meane agewith GCS <=12, 89% with PTA> 7 days	Consecutive admissions to inpateint rehab unit between 3/85 and 1/89 who completed 2 year with 5 year interviews
Walker, 2005(15)	(4) VA Polytrauma Network site Brain injury (rehab units)	Veterans-- Age 28.4, 91% male, 67% white, 73% injured in MVA, 6% penetrating injuries	Inclusion: consecutively admitted patients with moderate to severe TBI , veteran,cognitve function core greater than/equal to 5 (Rancho Los Amigos Scale

OTHER INJURIES

APPENDIX E, EVIDENCE TABLE 1. Studies on patient factors associated with polytrauma outcomes (Key Question 4)

Author, Year (ref.)	N enrolled, Tx v. controls	Exposure of interest	Control group: Comparator to exposure of interest	Pain-related outcomes measured	Timing of Outcomes	Is pain outcome a main outcome in
Hoffman, 2007(11)	146 subjects	n/a	n/a	2 item bodily pain of SF36	1 year	Yes
Lippert-Gruner, 2007(12)	49:28 w. severe TBI and 21 with severe TBI and additional injuries	TBI with additional injuries	TBI alone	SF 36--Bodily Pain/function	6 & 12 months	No
Masson, 1996(13)	Cases: 231 pts. W. TBI ; 80 lower limb injury pt. Controls	n/a	n/a	self report of headache and other pain	5 yrs after injury	No
Olver, 1996(14)	103	---	---	headaches	5 yrs after injury	No
Walker, 2005(15)	109	n/a	n/a	headache frequency, location, type, degree of incapacitation, headache density	6 & 12 months	Yes

OTHER INJURIES

APPENDIX E, EVIDENCE TABLE 1. Studies on patient factors associated with polytrauma outcomes (Key Question 4)

Author, Year (ref.)	Are results stratified or adjusted for polytrauma	Analytic method	Variables adjusted for in analysis or stratification
Hoffman, 2007(11)	yes--number of injuries	multivariate regression	Demographics, # and type of injuries, fuctional status at rehab discharge, baseline depression
Lippert-Gruner, 2007(12)	No	descriptive	None
Masson, 1996(13)	Yes	bivariate comparisons	Stratified by head injury severity
Olver, 1996(14)	No	bivariate comparisons	None
Walker, 2005(15)	All polytrauma patients	primarily bivariate, between group comparisons	----

OTHER
INJURIES

APPENDIX E, EVIDENCE TABLE 1. Studies on patient factors associated with polytrauma outcomes (Key Question 4)

Author, Year (ref.)	Results	Quality rating
Hoffman, 2007(11)	At one year, 74% of patients have pain, and 55% have functional interference . Baseline Glasgow Coma Scale score was not associated with pain status one year after injury. Pain one year after injury was significantly associated with being female and non-white. Being non-white and depression remained significantly associated with reports of pain at one year in a multivariate regression model (taking other factors into account).	Good
Lippert-Gruner, 2007(12)	No difference in bodily pain according to whether pt had additional injuries in addition to TBI	Poor
Masson, 1996(13)	The prevalence of headache was 44-54%, significantly greater than 16% in a comparison group with lower limb injury but no TBI. Headache and other pain prevalence is not significantly associated with head injury severity	Fair
Olver, 1996(14)	Headache prevalence increased from 31% at 2 yrs to 42% at 5 yrs	Poor
Walker, 2005(15)	Nearly 38% (41/109) of patients had acute headache symptoms; most often in a frontal location (20/41), most often of daily frequency (31/41) and showing no relation to injury severity, emotional, or demographic variable. Among patients with headaches at admission, 54% reported persistent headache symptoms at six months, and of this group, 96% still had headaches at 12 months. Headache improvement was associated with less anxiety and depression at 6 month followup.	Fair

OTHER INJURIES

APPENDIX E, EVIDENCE TABLE 1. Studies on patient factors associated with polytrauma outcomes (Key Question 4)

Author, Year (ref.)	Title	Topic area	Study Design	Sample: All polytrauma patients, majority, or just included?	Aims
Brenneman, 1997(16)	Long-term outcomes in open pelvic fractures	Orthopedic injuries	Cohort-retrospective	All	To document the injury characteristics, complications, and outcomes of trauma victims with an open pelvic fracture. We directed particular attention to two interventions under the control of trauma surgeons: blood transfusion and the use of a diverting colostomy. We also focused on 3 outcomes that occur only after the patient has left the trauma center: functional status, overall health perception, and return to work.

APPENDIX E, EVIDENCE TABLE 1. Studies on patient factors associated with polytrauma outcomes (Key Question 4)

Author, Year (ref.)	Setting	Sample demographics and other characteristics (include average time since injury at study baseline, if applicable)	Inclusion/exclusion criteria
Brenneman, 1997(16)	Sunnybrook Health Science Centre (SHC) is an adult regional trauma unit that treats mostly patients with blunt trauma (90%); 1987-1995	Patients with open fractures, n=44 Mean age 30, range 15-46 75% male Mechanism of injury: 27% motorcycle crash, 25% pedestrian, 21% motor vehicle crash Mean ISS 31, range 10-75 Patients with closed fractures - n=1,135 Mean age 39, range 12-93 57% male Mechanism of injury: 57% motor vehicle crash, 19% pedestrian Mean ISS 30, range 5-75 Major risk factors for open pelvic fracture: typical patient was a young male, frequently involved in a motorcycle crash, and more likely to have a severe unstable pelvic ring fracture.	All multiple system blunt trauma victims with a pelvic fracture admitted between Jan 1987 - July 1995 classifed as having either open or closed fractures.

APPENDIX E, EVIDENCE TABLE 1. Studies on patient factors associated with polytrauma outcomes (Key Question 4)

Author, Year (ref.)	N enrolled, Tx v. controls	Exposure of interest	Control group: Comparator to exposure of interest	Pain-related outcomes measured	Timing of Outcomes	Is pain outcome a main outcome in
Brenneman, 1997(16)	27 of 33 long-term survivors were available for followup	Open pelvic fractures	Closed pelvic fractures	Long-term survivors of an open pelvic fracture were assessed by phone interview using SF-36 and FIM. Additional Qs were on patient's employment, sexual functioning, and bowel and bladder function. Global health assessment, scale 0-100.	Mean followup 4 years after injury	Yes

APPENDIX E, EVIDENCE TABLE 1. Studies on patient factors associated with polytrauma outcomes (Key Question 4)

Author, Year (ref.)	Are results stratified or adjusted for polytrauma	Analytic method	Variables adjusted for in analysis or stratification
Brenneman, 1997(16)	All polytrauma	Comparison of means	None

APPENDIX E, EVIDENCE TABLE 1. Studies on patient factors associated with polytrauma outcomes (Key Question 4)

Author, Year (ref.)	Results	Quality rating
Brenneman, 1997(16)	SF-36 subscale mean score, open fractures (n=27) v. closed fractures (n=84) Bodily pain: 55.6 v. 66.1, p =ns Concludes: Patients with open pelvic fractures need to be treated with massive blood transfusions and often require a colostomy. They are frequently left with chronic pain and residual disabilities in physical functioning and physical roles, and many remain unemployed years after injury.	Fair

APPENDIX E, EVIDENCE TABLE 1. Studies on patient factors associated with polytrauma outcomes (Key Question 4)

Author, Year (ref.)	Title	Topic area	Study Design	Sample: All polytrauma patients, majority, or just included?	Aims
Hebert, 2000(17)	The effect of polytrauma in persons with traumatic spine injury. A prospective database of spine fractures	Orthopedic injuries: spine injury	Cohort-prospective	Majority.	1) to attempt to define predictors of injury severity in patients who sustain traumatic spinal injury; 2) to identify immediate, early, and late outcomes that are associated with severe or multiple injuries in this population. A 2nd objective was to determine whether one particular type of associate injury or region of injury is most predictive of outcome in these patients. Hypothesis: a higher severity of associated injuries adversely affects outcome in patients with traumatic spine injuries.

APPENDIX E, EVIDENCE TABLE 1. Studies on patient factors associated with polytrauma outcomes (Key Question 4)

Author, Year (ref.)	Setting	Sample demographics and other characteristics (include average time since injury at study baseline, if applicable)	Inclusion/exclusion criteria
Hebert, 2000(17)	Single hospital, all consecutive patients with traumatic spine injury; 1983-1992	patients with traumatic spine injury Mean age 32 71.7% male Mean ISS score 17.3 (range 4-75) Most common causes of injury: 58.9% MVA 17.6% sport or recreational injury 35.3% of patients had neurologic impairment. 71.7% of patients had polytrauma	Database of 830 spine trauma patients admitted consecutively to Univ of Alberta Hospital btw 1983-1992. Traumatic spine injury: spine fracture, dislocation, or subluxation, with or without neural injury. Excludes pathologic fracture without trauma, soft tissue or ligamentous injury without radiographically identified spine abnormality, and atraumatic injury. Excluded patients with only a minor transverse or spinous process fracture.

APPENDIX E, EVIDENCE TABLE 1. Studies on patient factors associated with polytrauma outcomes (Key Question 4)

Author, Year (ref.)	N enrolled, Tx v. controls	Exposure of interest	Control group: Comparator to exposure of interest	Pain-related outcomes measured	Timing of Outcomes	Is pain outcome a main outcome in
Hebert, 2000(17)	830	Severity of injury, quanitified by using AIS and ISS	---	Immediate outcomes: Neurologic impairment Loss of consciousness, low cervical injury, thoracic injury, multiple noncontinguous fracture, mixed fracture Early outcomes: early complications, complications requiring surgery, surgical treatment, death in hospital Late outcomes: no return to work at year 2, incapacitating pain year 1 2, incapacitating pain year 2. Only the late outcomes are abstracted here.	Immediate, early, up to 1 or 2 years	Yes

APPENDIX E, EVIDENCE TABLE 1. Studies on patient factors associated with polytrauma outcomes (Key Question 4)

Author, Year (ref.)	Are results stratified or adjusted for polytrauma	Analytic method	Variables adjusted for in analysis or stratification
Hebert, 2000(17)	No	Pearson's correlation coefficient. General factorial analysis of variance of nominal data with ISS as the dependent variable. Multiple linear regression for the association of each AIS region to FIM scores at discharge, 1 year, and 2 yrs after injury	Not reported

APPENDIX E, EVIDENCE TABLE 1. Studies on patient factors associated with polytrauma outcomes (Key Question 4)

Author, Year (ref.)	Results	Quality rating
Hebert, 2000[17]	Late outcomes: ISS had a significant negative correlation with FIM score at discharge, 1 year, and 2 years after injury. With stepwise linear regression, the AIS region accounting for most of the variance in FIM score was the spine (R2 0.383 at discharge, 0.429 at 1 year, 0.338 at 2 years) followed by the thorax at 1 year (R2 change, 0.005). 66% of patients returned to work by 2 years after injury. Those who did not return to work had significantly higher ISSs than those who returned to work: Mean ISS 22.65 v. 16.95, p<0.0001. Pts with higher ISS were more likely to have incapacitating pain v. occasional pain at 1 year (mean ISS 22.42 v. 14.99, p=0.001) and were more likely to have incapacitating pain (mean ISS 23.37) v. no pain (ISS 16.49) or occasional pain at 2 years (ISS 16.14), p=0.003. A letter by P.Anderson pointed out that defining polytrauma as an ISS of >9 is a much lower cutoff than that used in previous studies, and can reflect only moderate trauma to the spine, i.e., a spinal injury with a neurologic deficit and not truly multisystem trauma. A more commonly used value for the ISS is 18. Anderson also points out that the 39% lost to followup at 2 years may likely have better outcomes than those with permanent injuries who would continue with ongoing medical care or vocational rehabilitation. The FIM was designed to evaluate the neurologically impaired, especially quadriplegic patients, and might not have been useful in determining outcomes of extremity, chest, or abdominal trauma. Thus the results could have been biased to show that neurologic injury (i.e. severe spinal trauma) was the greatest predictor of outcome.	Fair

APPENDIX E, EVIDENCE TABLE 1. Studies on patient factors associated with polytrauma outcomes (Key Question 4)

Author, Year (ref.)	Title	Topic area	Study Design	Sample: All polytrauma patients, majority, or just included?	Aims
Tran, 2002(18)	Functional outcome of multiply injured patients with associated foot injury	Orthopedic injuries: foot injuries	Case control	All	To evaluate the ability of the AAOS lower extremity and foot and ankle questionnaire to discern a difference in outcome of polytrauma patients with and without foot injuries.

APPENDIX E, EVIDENCE TABLE 1. Studies on patient factors associated with polytrauma outcomes (Key Question 4)

Author, Year (ref.)	Setting	Sample demographics and other characteristics (include average time since injury at study baseline, if applicable)	Inclusion/exclusion criteria
Tran, 2002(18)	single institution trauma registry	Pts with v. without foot injuries: 85.7% v. 78.6% male Mean age = 29 v. 32 Mean ISS = 15 v. 17 Foot injuries included calcaneal fractures, Lisfranc fractures, talar fractures, midfoot fractures, and metatarsal fractures, with 2 pts suffering open injuries. Defined polytrauma as having an ISS >9. ISS scores >9 are associated with neurologic impairment or additional regions of injury. 71.7% of patients by this definition sustained polytrauma, with a mean ISS score of 20.56 +- 10.83. 28.3% had only spine fracture with no associated injury, with a mean ISS score of 8.95 +- 1.90.	Included 14 polytrauma patients with a foot injury, and 14 polytrauma patients without a foot injury. Each of these groups of patients were randomly selected from the institution's trauma registry. Inclusion criteria were: a minimal ISS of 12; survival of inintial injury with a minimum of 12 months of follow-up, and willingness to participate in a telephone survey.

APPENDIX E, EVIDENCE TABLE 1. Studies on patient factors associated with polytrauma outcomes (Key Question 4)

Author, Year (ref.)	N enrolled, Tx v. controls	Exposure of interest	Control group: Comparator to exposure of interest	Pain-related outcomes measured	Timing of Outcomes	Is pain outcome a main outcome in
Tran, 2002(18)	14 pts with foot injuries; 14 pts without foot injuries.	An AAOS lower extremity core questionnaire and foot and ankle; data gathered by chart review and telephone survey	Polytrauma without foot injuries	Chart review gathered data on age, sex, type of foot injury, and ISS. The questionnaire included the SF-36, and 3 lower extremity scores (physical health and pain, treatment expectations, and satisfaction with symptoms), and 2 foot and ankle scores (global foot and ankle scale and shoe comfort).	Not specified. Inclusion criteria required that patients have survived at least 12 months after injury.	Yes

APPENDIX E, EVIDENCE TABLE 1. Studies on patient factors associated with polytrauma outcomes (Key Question 4)

Author, Year (ref.)	Are results stratified or adjusted for polytrauma	Analytic method	Variables adjusted for in analysis or stratification
Tran, 2002(18)	No: all subjects PT	The results between the 2 groups were compared using a 2-tailed unpaired T-test with a $p < 0.05$ considered significant.	None

APPENDIX E, EVIDENCE TABLE 1. Studies on patient factors associated with polytrauma outcomes (Key Question 4)

Author, Year (ref.)	Results	Quality rating
Tran, 2002(18)	Patients with foot injuries had a dramatically lower physical function, role physical (a perception of their physical functioning), bodily pain, and social function scores compared to the control group. All 5 of the scales specific to lower extremity and foot and ankle questions were significantlly different, with lower physical health and pain scores, treatment expectation scores, and satisfaction with symptom scores, global foot and ankle scale scores, and shoe comfort scores, among patients with foot injuries. In 5 of the 10 SF-36 scores, patients in the foot injury group had significantly lower scores. With v. without foot injuries: Mean SF-36 score: Physical function 80.7 v. 38.9, $p<0.05$ Role-physical 87.5 v. 41.1, $p<0.05$ Bodily pain 81.9 v. 50.6, $p<0.05$ Social function 96.6 v. 67.9, $p<0.05$ Physical composite score 47.8 v. 30.8, $p<0.05$ In all 5 off the lower-extremity scores, the foot-injured group had lower scores than the control group: Physical health and pain: 83.3 v. 43.5, $p<0.05$ Treatment expectations: 83.8 v. 55.7, $p<0.05$ Satisfaction with symptoms: 4 v. 1.5, $p<0.05$ Global foot and ankle scale: 100 v. 57.6, $p<0.05$ Shoe comfort: 100 v. 18.9, $p<0.05$	Fair

APPENDIX E, EVIDENCE TABLE 1. Studies on patient factors associated with polytrauma outcomes (Key Question 4)

Author, Year (ref.)	Title	Topic area	Study Design	Sample: All polytrauma patients, majority, or just included?	Aims
Turchin, 1999(19)	Do foot injuries significantly affect the functional outcome of multiply injured patients?	Orthopedic injuries: foot injuries	Cohort study-Prospective, matched pair	All	1) To assess the functional outcome of a specific subgroup of trauma patients, that is, multiply injured patients with foot injuries. 2) To determine which measures are most appropriate for assessing the functional outcome of these patients.
Urquhart, 2006(20)	Outcomes of patients with orthopaedic trauma admitted to level 1 trauma centres	Orthopedic injuries	Cohort-prospective	Included: 2 of 3 subgroups have multiple injuries	To investigate the outcomes of patients admitted with a variety of orthopedic injuries to 2 adult Level 1 trauma centers in Victoria, Australia.

APPENDIX E, EVIDENCE TABLE 1. Studies on patient factors associated with polytrauma outcomes (Key Question 4)

Author, Year (ref.)	Setting	Sample demographics and other characteristics (include average time since injury at study baseline, if applicable)	Inclusion/exclusion criteria
Turchin, 1999(19)	University-affiliated Level 1 trauma center with a prospectively entered trauma database.	In 28 pts with foot injuries: 60.7% male (n=17 males; 11 females) Mean age 34 years (range 18-63); Mean ISS 25 (range 13-41); Mean hospital stay = 24 days; Mean ICU stay = 5 days; Mean duration of followup = 62 months Foot injuries were calcaneal fractures (n=13), talar fractures (n=6), Lisfranc fracture dislocations (n=4), other midfoot fractures (n=4), metatarsal fractures (n=8), and phalangeal fractures (n=2) In 28 pts without foot injuries: Mean age was 36 (range 16-70); Mean ISS 25 (range 13-41) Mean hospital stay = 25 days; Mean ICU stay = 7 days; Mean duration of followup = 69 months No significant btw-group differences in demographics.	28 multiply injured patients with foot injuries were identified in a prospectively entered trauma database. These patients could then be matched in a blinded fashion to multiply injured patients who did not have foot injuries but were of the same sex, and within 10 years of age, within 5 points of the ISS, and within 1 year of follow-up.
Urquhart, 2006(20)	Victorian Orthopedic Trauma Outcomes Registry - all pts with trauma admitted to the 2 adult Level 1 trauma centers in Victoria, Australia; August 2003-2004	893 completed the 6-month follow-up, out of 1181 eligible.	VOTOR trauma registry includes all pts with an orthopedic injury admitted over a 12 month period (Auguest 2003-2004) to the 2 adult Level 1 trauma centers in Victoria, Australia. Excludes patients that had a pathological fracture related to metastatic disease and/or an isolated orthopedic injury managed by another unit. Also excluded pts with a diagnosis of dementia or mental illness, or were less than 6 months post-injury.

APPENDIX E, EVIDENCE TABLE 1. Studies on patient factors associated with polytrauma outcomes (Key Question 4)

Author, Year (ref.)	N enrolled, Tx v. controls	Exposure of interest	Control group: Comparator to exposure of interest	Pain-related outcomes measured	Timing of Outcomes	Is pain outcome a main outcome in
Turchin, 1999(19)	28 with foot injuries; 28 without foot injuries	Polytrauma plus foot injuries; data gathered by telephone survey	Polytrauma wihout foot injuries Prospective matched pair analysis. Does not describe the other non-foot trauma injuries that the patients sustained, in order to qualify as "multiply injured".	Outcomes were determined by telephone survey. SF-36, a global health measure with 8 components: physical functioning, role physical, bodily pain, general health, vitality, social functioning, role emotional, and mental health. WOMAC, a disease-specific scale designed to measure status of patients with osteoarthritis of the lower extremity. 3 components: physical function, pain, and stiffness. Modified Boston Children's Hospital Grading System, a foot-and-ankle score for assessing patients with ankle arthrodeses. 2 components: pain, physical function (a 3rd, range of motion, could not be assessed by telephone, and was omitted).	2 years minimum. Mean followup 62 months. Cases and controls were matched on timing of followup (within 1 year of each other)	Yes
Urquhart, 2006(20)	659 pts with multiple orthopedic injuries (with no other injuries) 165 patients with single/multiple ortho injuries plus other injuries	1) Patients with multiple orthopedic injuries (with no other injuries 2) Patients with single/multiple orthopedic injuries and other injuries.	Patients with an isolated orthopedic injury, with no other injury	Pain, disability, SF12 assessed at 6 months post-injury by questionnaire. All patients were initially contacted by phone to complete the questoinnaires. Questoinnaires were mailed to patients who could not complete it at the time of the call.	6 months post-injury	Yes

APPENDIX E, EVIDENCE TABLE 1. Studies on patient factors associated with polytrauma outcomes (Key Question 4)

Author, Year (ref.)	Are results stratified or adjusted for polytrauma	Analytic method	Variables adjusted for in analysis or stratification
Turchin, 1999(19)	No: all subjects PT	2-tailed unpaired t tests to assess whether foot injureis affect the outcome of multiply injured patients. The correlation of the 3 outcome measures was assessed for both groups of patients to determine the relative usefulness of the scales.	None
Urquhart, 2006(20)	Yes	Mann-Whitny U-test to compare continuous variables, such as age, pain a- 6 months and SF12 physical and mental scores. Chi2 tests for associations between injury groups and categorical variables.	None

APPENDIX E, EVIDENCE TABLE 1. Studies on patient factors associated with polytrauma outcomes (Key Question 4)

Author, Year (ref.)	Results	Quality rating
Turchin, 1999(19)	Response rate to telephone survey not reported. The outcome of multiply injured patients with foot injuries was significantly worse than that of patients without foot injuries when using any of the 3 outcome measures. Patients with v. without foot injuries: Mean SF-36 score: 49 v. 66 (p=0.008) Mean total WOMAC score: 34 v. 13 (p=0.00007) Mean modified Boston Children's score: 634 v. 78 (p=0.001)	Fair
Urquhart, 2006(20)	Moderate/severe pain at 6 months was most frequent among pts with single/multiple ortho injuries plus other injuries (46.7%), compared with 36.9% of patients with multiple ortho (without other) injuries, and 32.5% of patietns with an isolated ortho injury. P<0.05 for differences between groups. MOderate/severe disability was more frequent among these groups in a similar pattern (52.7% v. 50.3% v. 44.1%, p<0.05 groups 2 and 3 v. 1), although the 2 groups with multiple injuries did not differ from each other. % not working at all post-injury was highest in the group with single/multiple ortho plus other injuries (42.5%), compared with multiple ortho injuries only (38.2%) and isolated injuries (18.8%). (p<0.05 group 1 differs from 2 and 3)	Fair

APPENDIX E, EVIDENCE TABLE 1. Studies on patient factors associated with polytrauma outcomes (Key Question 4)

Author, Year (ref.)	Title	Topic area	Study Design	Sample: All polytrauma patients, majority, or just included?	Aims
Zelle, 2005(21)	The impact of injuries below the knee joint on the long-term functional outcome following polytrauma	Orthopedic injuries: below-knee injuries	Cohort study	All	The purpose of the Hannover Rehab Study was to identify specific variables that are predictive of the long-term outcome following polytrauma. To evaluate the impact of injuries below the knee joint on the long-term functional outcome following polytrauma.
Anke, 1997(22)	Long-term prevalence of impairments and disabilities after multiple trauma.	long-term followup	Cohort-retrospective	All	To analyze the prevalence of impairments and disabilities after sever multiple trauma. Specifically, to address the following questions: To what extent is the injury-type and severity predictive of late impairment and disabilities? To what extent does the trauma cause changes in the quantity and quality of social networks? To what extent do demographic variables and impairments influence the ability to manage personal activities of daily living, nonwork activities, and work?

APPENDIX E, EVIDENCE TABLE 1. Studies on patient factors associated with polytrauma outcomes (Key Question 4)

Author, Year (ref.)	Setting	Sample demographics and other characteristics (include average time since injury at study baseline, if applicable)	Inclusion/exclusion criteria
Zelle, 2005(21)	Hannover Rehab Study: cohort study, Germany; 1973-1990	389 patients: 287 (74%) male Mean follow-up 17.3 +- 4.8 years Mean age 25.4 Mean ISS 20.2 Mean PTS 29.5	637 polytrauma patients who were treated at the study site between 1973-1990 were re-evaluated by a doctor or an outpatient basis. Patients were enrolled in the study by these criteria: -Polytrauma between 1973-1990 associated with one or more lower-extremity fractures. -Treatment at our level one trauma centre -Aged 3-60 at the time of injury -Minimum follow-up of at least 10 yrs 389 were eligble for the study - report suggests that all eligible were followed up.
Anke, 1997(22)	Ulleval Hospital in Oslo, Norway	70% male. Mean age at time of injury 33 +/-16 years. 71% had higher education. Among the subjects regularly working or studying at the time of injury, 14 blue-collar, 44 white collar (including 15 students). Mean ISS=25 (range 17-50).	*Inclusion*: All patients with severe multiple trauma; Age >=12 yrs; Admitted within 24 hours of injury to the department of surgery at the Ulleval Hospital in Oslo during 1990; ISS>16. *Exclusion*: <12 yrs (n=3); Dead (n=5); Living abroad (n=9); Unknown address (n=5); Subsequent serious injury (n=1).

APPENDIX E, EVIDENCE TABLE 1. Studies on patient factors associated with polytrauma outcomes (Key Question 4)

Author, Year (ref.)	N enrolled, Tx v. controls	Exposure of interest	Control group: Comparator to exposure of interest	Pain-related outcomes measured	Timing of Outcomes	Is pain outcome a main outcome in
Zelle, 2005(21)	389	Injuries below the knee joint	Injuries above the knee joint	patients treated at trauma center betw 1973-1990 were re-evaluated by a doctor on an outpatient basis, usgin a standardized self-administered patient questionniare and a standardised physical exam of the injured body regions, including the modified Karlstrom-Olerud score, Lysholm score, range of motion of hip, knee, and ankle joint, weight bearing status of the injured lower-extremity, persistent pain of the injured lower-extremity, and gait. General outcomes measured include the Hannover score for polytrauma outcome (HASPOC), 12-item short-form health survey (SF-12), Tegner activity score, and the inability to work. Ability to work at followup was only	10+ years post injury	No, but part as functional status scale
Anke, 1997(22)	N enrolled=69	Abbreviated Injury Scale; Demographic variables; Social network questionnaire; Occurrence of impairments and disabilities	[compared to general population]	Social network; Impairments; Disabilities	35 +/-4 months post injury	Yes

APPENDIX E, EVIDENCE TABLE 1. Studies on patient factors associated with polytrauma outcomes (Key Question 4)

Author, Year (ref.)	Are results stratified or adjusted for polytrauma	Analytic method	Variables adjusted for in analysis or stratification
Zelle, 2005(21)	All polytrauma patients	3 groups were compared, based on pattern of injury: 1) injured lower extremities with fractures above knee joint; 2) fractures below the knee joint but without associated unilateral fractures above knee joint; 3) combined fractures above and below the knee joint. General outcomes compared 2 groups: 1) fractures below the knee joint on at least one side (including combined injuries); 2) patients with lower-extremity fractures solely above the knee joint. Logistic regression for each outcome measurement for below-knee group,	Logistic regression adjusted for age, gender, and ISS - these variables were significantly different between patients with injuries above and below knee.
Anke, 1997(22)	no, all patients included are polytrauma patients	Ror comparisons of groups of data simple cross tabulations were performed Chi-Squared test or Fischer's exact test. Correlations were analyzed with Spearman's P. The Mann-Whitney nonparametric two-sample test was used to analyze differences in medians. The sign test was used to analyze the changes in activity preferences. Values of p of <= 0.05 were considered statistically significant.	None

APPENDIX E, EVIDENCE TABLE 1. Studies on patient factors associated with polytrauma outcomes (Key Question 4)

Author, Year (ref.)	Results	Quality rating
Zelle, 2005(21)	Below knee (n=156) v. combined injuries (n=170): Persistent pain: 45.5% v. 58.8%, p=0.016 Above knee (n=183) v. below knee (n=156): Persistent pain 39.3% v. 45.5%, p=0.252 Above knee (n=183) v. combined injuries (n=170): Persistent pain 39.3% v. 38.8%, p<0.0005 Inability to work: Fractures below the knee joint v. above knee joint: OR 2.21 (1.10-4.43) concludes: Fractures below the knee joint have a significant impact on the functional recovery following polytrauma.	Good
Anke, 1997(22)	Associations between all Leisure Disability (LD) (n=51) & Vocational Disability (VD) (n=11) and other factors: Age LD=ns; VD=p<0.01; Blue/white-collar work LD=ns; VD=p<0.05. Decrease of social network quantity LD=ns; VD=p<0.05; Decrease in social network quality LD=ns; VD=p<0.01; Injury severity score LD=ns; VD=p<0.05. Cognitive impairment LD=ns; VD=p<0.05; Physical impairment LD=p<0.01; VD=ns; Pain LD=p<0.05; VD=ns. Numbers of lost leisure activities LD=N/A; VD=p<0.05.	Fair

APPENDIX E, EVIDENCE TABLE 1. Studies on patient factors associated with polytrauma outcomes (Key Question 4)

Author, Year (ref.)	Title	Topic area	Study Design	Sample: All polytrauma patients, majority, or just included?	Aims
Brenneman, 1997(23)	Long-term outcomes in blunt trauma: who goes back to work?	long-term followup	Cohort-prospective	Not specified, mean ISS=25	To compare the characteristics of patients who do and do not return to work after blunt trauma.
Dimopoulou, 2004(24)	Health-related quality of life and disability in survivors of multiple trauma one year after intensive care unit discharge.	long-term followup	Cohort-prospective	All	To evaluate health-related quality of life and disability in multiple-trauma patients requiring intensive care unit management.
Fitzharris, 2007(25)	General Health Status and Function al Disability Following Injury in Traffic Crashes	long-term followup, car accidents	Cohort-prospective	Included	To examine general health status and functional disability at 2 months and 6-8 months post-crash

APPENDIX E, EVIDENCE TABLE 1. Studies on patient factors associated with polytrauma outcomes (Key Question 4)

Author, Year (ref.)	Setting	Sample demographics and other characteristics (include average time since injury at study baseline, if applicable)	Inclusion/exclusion criteria
Brenneman, 1997(23)	Sunnybrook Health Science Center (a regional trauma unit that admits the majority of adult multiple system trauma patients in Toronto and surrounding areas in the province of Ontario Canada).	65% male. Mean age=37. Mean ISS=25.	*Inclusion:* Discharged from the hospital between July 1994 and June of 1995. *Exclusion:* ISS<=10; Patients who left with incapacitating head injuries.
Dimopoulou, 2004(24)	A tertiary teaching hospital in Athens , Greece.	74% male. Mean age=31. Mean 1SS=22 (11-41)	*Inclusion:* all consecutive multiple-trauma patients admitted in the ICU during the period of 1999-2000. *Exclusion:* not described
Fitzharris, 2007(25)	A major trauma center and 2 metropolitan teaching hospitals in Victoria, Australia	35 males, 27 females Mean age 35.3 (males), 38.7 (females) % employed; 100% males, 96.3% females Mean ISS: 9.5 males, 11.1 females; 10.2 total % with major trauma, i.e. ISS >15: 14.3% males, 18.5 females; 16.1% total 48% had fracture of lower extremity, and 61.3% had fracture of upper extremity. More males than females had fractures of lower leg (37.1% v. 14.8%, p<0.05).	Healthy adults aged 18-59 admitted to hospitals following involvement in a road traffic crash. Excluded those with moderate-severe head injury and spinal cord injury. Unclear whether analysis included all eligible patients, or a sample (those with data from all 3 timepoints).

APPENDIX E, EVIDENCE TABLE 1. Studies on patient factors associated with polytrauma outcomes (Key Question 4)

Author, Year (ref.)	N enrolled, Tx v. controls	Exposure of interest	Control group: Comparator to exposure of interest	Pain-related outcomes measured	Timing of Outcomes	Is pain outcome a main outcome in
Brenneman, 1997(23)	N enrolled = 195	Questionnaire at time of discharge and phone interview 1 yr post injury.	general population	Return to work (RTW)	1 yr post injury	No
Dimopoulou, 2004(24)	N eligible patients=117. N enrolled= 87	Questionnaires at 1 yr post injury	general population	Nottingham Health Profile, Glasgow Outcome Scale and Rosser Disability Scale	1 yr post injury	No
Fitzharris, 2007(25)	62 adults completed interviews prior to discharge and at 2 and 8 months post-discharge	traffic accident	differences over time; differences by gender	Self-reported pain, using 100-pt VAS, assessed by interviews on 3 occasions: discharge, 2-months and 8 months post-discharge.	2 months and 8 months post-discharge	Yes

APPENDIX E, EVIDENCE TABLE 1. Studies on patient factors associated with polytrauma outcomes (Key Question 4)

Author, Year (ref.)	Are results stratified or adjusted for polytrauma	Analytic method	Variables adjusted for in analysis or stratification
Brenneman, 1997(23)	All polytrauma patients	Two regression models	None
Dimopoulou, 2004(24)	All polytrauma patients	Normality of the distributions of variables was examined using the Komogorov-Smirnov test. Relationships between variables were analyzed by Spearman's correlation coefficient. To identify factors predicting HRqoL and disability, logistic regression analysis was performed.	None
Fitzharris, 2007(25)	No	Comparisons between males and females were made using chi-square tests, and 2way repeated measures ANOVA using a mixed design 3(time) x2 (gender) with planned comparisons between timepoint scores.	Gender, and time

APPENDIX E, EVIDENCE TABLE 1. Studies on patient factors associated with polytrauma outcomes (Key Question 4)

Author, Year (ref.)	Results	Quality rating
Brenneman, 1997(23)	Factors associated with RTW: younger age (p<0.0001); professional employment (p<0.0001); lower ISS (p<0.001).	Fair
Dimopoulou, 2004(24)	Factors associated with lower score on Nottingham Health Profile: higher ISS (p=0.008) & head injury (p=0.038). Factors associated with disability (Rosser Disability Scale): higher ISS (p=0.004) & head injury (0.004)	Fair
Fitzharris, 2007(25)	There were no significant differences by gender in self-reported pain (100-pt VAS scale) at 8 months post-discharge. At 2 months post-discharge, the % reporting Zero pain was 11.4% of males, and 3.7% of females. At 8 months: 20% of males, 22% of females.	Fair

APPENDIX E, EVIDENCE TABLE 1. Studies on patient factors associated with polytrauma outcomes (Key Question 4)

Author, Year (ref.)	Title	Topic area	Study Design	Sample: All polytrauma patients, majority, or just included?	Aims
Holtslag, 2007(26)	Determinants of long-term functional consequences after major trauma.	long-term followup	Cohort-prospective	Majority	To quantify the prevalence and determinants of the functional outcome of severely injured patients, studying the influence of sociodemographic, injury-related factors, and of physical factors.

APPENDIX E, EVIDENCE TABLE 1. Studies on patient factors associated with polytrauma outcomes (Key Question 4)

Author, Year (ref.)	Setting	Sample demographics and other characteristics (include average time since injury at study baseline, if applicable)	Inclusion/exclusion criteria
Holtslag, 2007(26)	University Medical Center Utrecht, 1 of the 10 Level I trauma hospitals in the Netherlands, serving a catchment area with population if 1.1 million. Utrecht is an urbanized area in the center of the Netherlands with a population density of 813 inhabitants per square kilometer.	74% male (Mean age= 36.6) 36% female (Mean age=41.0 years)	*Inclusion:* Severely injured patients referred from emergency care during 1999 and 2000; ISS>16. *Exclusions:* Age<16

APPENDIX E, EVIDENCE TABLE 1. Studies on patient factors associated with polytrauma outcomes (Key Question 4)

Author, Year (ref.)	N enrolled, Tx v. controls	Exposure of interest	Control group: Comparator to exposure of interest	Pain-related outcomes measured	Timing of Outcomes	Is pain outcome a main outcome in
Holtslag, 2007(26)	N eligible patients=359; N enrolled=311	self-administered questionnaires	general Dutch population	Health status as measured by EQ-5D; Disability as measured by Glasgow Outcome Scale; Head injury symptom checklist (HISC); Comorbidity using health and labor questionnaire from which depression was excluded.	randomized range of 12 to 28 months after trauma	only as part of EQ-5D

APPENDIX E, EVIDENCE TABLE 1. Studies on patient factors associated with polytrauma outcomes (Key Question 4)

Author, Year (ref.)	Are results stratified or adjusted for polytrauma	Analytic method	Variables adjusted for in analysis or stratification
Holtslag, 2007(26)	comorbidity is analyzed as a predictor of outcomes	The outcomes of the five individual EZ dimensions were dichotomized as no problems vs. some or severe problems. Also dichotomized, symptoms of cognitive yes/no as well as functional limitations yes/no. Other determinants divided into two groups were gender, age, injury severity, localization of injury, education, bmi, sports activities before injury, depression and comorbidity. dichotomized determinants and dichotomous outcomes were tested with Pearson Chi-Squared test; between dichotomized determinants and linear outcomes Mann-Whitney U test. the adjusted impact of the potential determinants on all dichotomized outcome variables was determined by mans of multivariate logistic regression analyses.	no

APPENDIX E, EVIDENCE TABLE 1. Studies on patient factors associated with polytrauma outcomes (Key Question 4)

Author, Year (ref.)	Results	Quality rating
Holtslag, 2007(26)	Factors associated with poor Glasgow Outcome Scale (general disability) as significant according to Chi-Squared test: aged 55 or older; Brain injury; Spinal cord injury; Low educational level; Comorbidity. Factors associates with lower EQ (quality of life) scores: Education (p<0.05); Comorbidity (p<0.05); Education (p<0.05); Brain Injury (p<0.05); Spinal cor injury and lower extremity injury (p<0.001).	Fair

APPENDIX E, EVIDENCE TABLE 1. Studies on patient factors associated with polytrauma outcomes (Key Question 4)

Author, Year (ref.)	Title	Topic area	Study Design	Sample: All polytrauma patients, majority, or just included?	Aims
MacKenzie, 1998(27)	Return to work following injury: the role of economic, social and job-related factors.	long-term followup	Cohort-prospective	Included	To examine factors influencing return to work for severe fracture to the lower extremities.
Meerding, 2004(28)	Distribution and determinants of health and work status in a comprehensive population of injury patients.	long-term followup	Cohort-prospective	Included	To answer the following questions: How are the levels of functioning and work status distributed across patient groups in the first year after injury? How does the health status of injury patients compare with the general population? What personal, injury and health care factors are predictive for levels of functioning and work status?

APPENDIX E, EVIDENCE TABLE 1. Studies on patient factors associated with polytrauma outcomes (Key Question 4)

Author, Year (ref.)	Setting	Sample demographics and other characteristics (include average time since injury at study baseline, if applicable)	Inclusion/exclusion criteria
MacKenzie, 1998(27)	Patients recruited from three level-1 trauma centers: Harborview medical Center (Seattle, WA), the R Adams Cowley Shock Trauma Center (Baltimore, MD) and Vanderbilt University Medical Center (Nashville, TN)	Aged 18 to 64, worked full time before the injury	*Inclusion:* Patients admitted for treatment of blunt, unilateral lower extremity fracture distal or including the acetabulum. *Exclusions* : patellar fractures and minor foot fractures; Patients who recieved definitive care outside the trauma center; Had a major neurologic injury, an unstable spinal cord injury, or an upper extremity injury that precluded the use of crutches or walker; Had a psychiatric illness; Had lower extremity fracture secondary illness; No English spoken; Did not live in the trauma center's catchments area; On active military duty
Meerding, 2004(28)	Hospital emergency departments of the Dutch Injury Surveillance System. 17 hospitals in the Netherlands (approx. 15% coverage) These hospitals are geographically spread across the country; include both academic and nonacademic hospitals, trauma centers, and nontrauma centers; and cover representative amounts to urban and rural populations.	54% Male. 72.6% <65yrs.	*Inclusion:* Visited one of the hospital emergency department in the system with an injury. *Exclusion:* Age<15; Victims of self-inflicted injury; Institutionalized persons.

APPENDIX E, EVIDENCE TABLE 1. Studies on patient factors associated with polytrauma outcomes (Key Question 4)

Author, Year (ref.)	N enrolled, Tx v. controls	Exposure of interest	Control group: Comparator to exposure of interest	Pain-related outcomes measured	Timing of Outcomes	Is pain outcome a **main** outcome in
MacKenzie, 1998(27)	N elegible=341; N enrolled=312.	patient interview and evaluation by physical therapist	general population	Time in days from injury to first time the study participant returned to work	1 yr post injury	No
Meerding, 2004(28)	N eligible=4639. N enrolled=1806.	questionnaire (postal) EuroQuol (EQ-5D) and EQ-5D+ (for cognitive function) as well as return to work status	EuroQol data from the Swedish general population	responses to EQ5+ as well as return to work status	2 mo, 5 mo and 9 mo after injury	pain as part of functioning and health measured by EQ5+ as well as return to work status

APPENDIX E, EVIDENCE TABLE 1. Studies on patient factors associated with polytrauma outcomes (Key Question 4)

Author, Year (ref.)	Are results stratified or adjusted for polytrauma	Analytic method	Variables adjusted for in analysis or stratification
MacKenzie, 1998(27)	No	Log-rank test used to test the association between the cumulative probability of RTW and each risk factor considered one at a time. A cox proport onal hazards regression model was used to estimate the combined effect of multiple risk factors while accounting for the effect of pain and impairments.	Effect of impairment; Pain
Meerding, 2004(28)	Yes	A nonresponce analysis was performed by forward stepwise multivariate logistic regression separate for the 2, 5 and nine month measurements. Regression analyses on the weighted data of each follow-up measurements. The sociodemographic and injury-related characteristics were tested as significant predictors of functional outcome and wok status in forward-step multivariate regression analyses. they were all entered as categorical variables.	Age, Sex, Education level,

APPENDIX E, EVIDENCE TABLE 1. Studies on patient factors associated with polytrauma outcomes (Key Question 4)

Author, Year (ref.)	Results	Quality rating
MacKenzie, 1998(27)	Factors associated with higher rates of RTW (P<0.05) : Higher levels of education, Family incomes above 125% of the federal poverty level, High levels of social support (particularly in terms of available practical assistance), Absence of alcoholism, Job stability, Job flexibility, White-collar employment, Employment in jobs with low physical demands. Both the receipt of workers' compensation and involvement with the legal system were associated with lower rates of RTW. Pain was highly correlated with impairment.	Good
Meerding, 2004(28)	Number of injuries is a determinant of health and work status. Factors associated with poor QoL (EQ-5D): Age (P<0.0001); Sex (P<0.001); LOS times type of injury (p<0.05); Education(P<0.01). Factors Associated with RTW: Hospital LOS (p<0.0001); Admittance to ICU (p<0.05); Education (P<0.01).	Good

APPENDIX E, EVIDENCE TABLE 1. Studies on patient factors associated with polytrauma outcomes (Key Question 4)

Author, Year (ref.)	Title	Topic area	Study Design	Sample: All polytrauma patients, majority, or just included?	Aims
Mkandawire, 2002(29)	Musculoskeletal recovery 5 years after severe injury: long term problems are common.	long-term followup	Cohort-prospective	Majority	To report the incidence of functional problems and pain for different types of injuries: shoulder girdle, upper limb, lower limb and pelvic injuries.
Soberg, 2007(30)	Long-term multidimensional functional consequences of severe multiple injuries two years after trauma: a prospective longitudinal cohort study	long-term followup	Cohort study-Prospective	All	To explore the functional health status and disease burden of patients with severe multiple injuries from after the return home until 2 years after injury.

APPENDIX E, EVIDENCE TABLE 1. Studies on patient factors associated with polytrauma outcomes (Key Question 4)

Author, Year (ref.)	Setting	Sample demographics and other characteristics (include average time since injury at study baseline, if applicable)	Inclusion/exclusion criteria
Mkandawire, 2002(29)	Sixteen hospitals in a large geographical area, Mersey Region and North Wales.	Mean age=36.5. All were severely injured "usually involving several body regions"	*Inclusion:* In a 12 month period in 1989-1990 patients discharged alive from a hospital having sustained severe injuries. *Exclusions:* Reside outside an area around the research centre, where follow-up appointments at hospital or home visits could feasibly be arranged.
Soberg, 2007(30)	Ulleval University Hospital in Oslo, Norway, a trauma referral center with a population base of nearly 2.5 million people and approximately 900 trauma team activations each year.	83% male. Mean age=35.3; 72% high school or higher; 55% married or living with partner; 63% blue collar workers	*Inclusion:* Aged 18 -67; New Injury Severity Score (NISS)>=16; At least two injuries classified in the abbreviated Injury Severity Scale (AIS) injury scoring system. *Exclusion:* Former multiple injuries; Burn injuries only; Substance addiction; Severe psychological disease registered in medical record; Aphasia; Insufficient command of the Norwegian language.

APPENDIX E, EVIDENCE TABLE 1. Studies on patient factors associated with polytrauma outcomes (Key Question 4)

Author, Year (ref.)	N enrolled, Tx v. controls	Exposure of interest	Control group: Comparator to exposure of interest	Pain-related outcomes measured	Timing of Outcomes	Is pain outcome a main outcome in
Mkandawire, 2002(29)	N enrolled =158	disability was assessed and graded by an assessor after an interview and detailed physical examination using the Bull Disability Scale. Pain was graded by the patient according to undefined categories, none, mild, moderate or severe	none; compared to patients from EPITOME study not studied in this study	Single assessment of functional disability and pain	5 years post injury	Yes
Soberg, 2007(30)	N elegible=169. N enrolled=101.	Questionnaires including the following instruments: SF-36; WHODAS II; COG scale (plus demographic data)	none; compared to general population scores or patients from MacKenzie study	SF-36: Physical functioning; Role physical; Bodily pain; General health; Vitality; Social functioning; Role emotional; Mental health, COG, WHODAS II also injuries were rated by approved trauma registrar for severity (1-6) and location (head/neck; face; chest; abdomen/pelvic content; extremities; external)	at time of injury upon discharge from hospital, 1yr post injury & 2yr post injury	Yes

APPENDIX E, EVIDENCE TABLE 1. Studies on patient factors associated with polytrauma outcomes (Key Question 4)

Author, Year (ref.)	Are results stratified or adjusted for polytrauma	Analytic method	Variables adjusted for in analysis or stratification
Mkandawire, 2002(29)	Yes; single fractures compared to multiple fractures	descriptive statistics	None
Soberg, 2007(30)	All polytrauma patients, compared against general population	Descriptive statistics; for non-parametric data: chi-squared tests, spearman's p or Pearson's r. for parametric data t tests and ANOVA. For multiple comparisons, Bonferroini correction	Yes

APPENDIX E, EVIDENCE TABLE 1. Studies on patient factors associated with polytrauma outcomes (Key Question 4)

Author, Year (ref.)	Results	Quality rating
Mkandawire, 2002(29)	44% of patients with single fractures had residual disability. 90% of patients with multiple fractures had residual disability.	Fair
Soberg, 2007(30)	Head injury patients scored an average of 13.7 points worse on COG scale at 2 yr post injury (p=0.002). 2 years post injury the most important predictor variable for role physical were physical functioning both shortly after return home and 1 yr after injury (p<0.00001). Variables at 1 year after injury that predict role physical at 2 years were profession (p=0.019), social functioning (p=0.047) and physical functioning (p<0.001). For WHODAS II (disability rating) predictors for a low disability rating at year 2 were: time from injury to return home (p=0.001), social functioning (p<0.001) and physical functioning(p=0.003); Predictors at year 1 were: profession(p=0.017), injury severity (p=0.0001), bodily pain (p=0.042), social functioning (p=0.030), physical functioning (p<0.001) and cognitive function	Good

APPENDIX E, EVIDENCE TABLE 1. Studies on patient factors associated with polytrauma outcomes (Key Question 4)

Author, Year (ref.)	Title	Topic area	Study Design	Sample: All polytrauma patients, majority, or just included?	Aims
Vles, 2005(31)	Prevalence and determinants of disabilities and return to work after major trauma.	long-term followup	Cohort-prospective	Included	to assess the prevalence and determinants of disabilities and return to work after severe injury
Dougherty, 1999(32)	Long-term Follow-up Study of Bilateral Above the Knee Amputees from the vietnam War	Amputation, quality of life	Cohort study-- retrospective	All	To document long-term outcomes for pts. Who had a bilateral above the knee amputatoin during the vietnam war
Dougherty, 2001(33)	Transtibial amputees from the Vietnam War. Twenty-eight-year follow-up	Amputation, transtibial headache veteran	Cohort-- retrospective	Majority	To compare long-term functional outcome btw 2 groups: 1) An isolated amputation 2) Amputation and at least 1 other major injury All had transtibial amputation.
Frink, 2007(34)	Long term results of compartment syndrome of the lower limb in polytraumatized patients	KQ2,4: compartment syndrome, non-veteran	Cohort study-- retrospective	Majority	Examine outcome of cmpartment syndrome of lower limb in patients with multiple injuries versus patients with single injury p. 608

APPENDIX E, EVIDENCE TABLE 1. Studies on patient factors associated with polytrauma outcomes (Key Question 4)

Author, Year (ref.)	Setting	Sample demographics and other characteristics (include average time since injury at study baseline, if applicable)	Inclusion/exclusion criteria
Vles, 2005(31)	St. Elisabeth Hospital in Tilburg, the Netherlands, one of the 10 regional Level I trauma centers in the Netherlands.	81% male; mean age=33; Mean ISS=23. 19% female; Mean age=37; Mean ISS of 23.	*Inclusion:* Trauma patient admitted to St. Elisabeth Hospital between Jan 1996 and Jan 1999 with an ISS >=16 *Exclusion:* not reported
Dougherty, 1999(32)	pts. Seen in a single hospital during vietnam war. Pts. Were contacted years later and asked to complete this study.	Veterans mean=47.8 a time of survey(27.5 yrs after injury)91% married	only inclusion is having a apecific type of surgery at a certain hospital during the vietnam war
Dougherty, 2001(33)	Retrospective chart review of pts seen for transtibial amputation during the Vietnam War. These pts were then recontacted an avg of 28 years later, and asked to complete questionnaires	Veterans, race not specified Group 1 v. Group 2: Mean age 48.9 v. 48.1 Employed 100% v. 98% Married 93% v. 98% Kids 82% v. 84% History psych Tx = 21% v. 50%	Underwent transtibial amputation at a specific hospital during Vietnam war. only subset used to match the control group, based on age
Frink, 2007(34)	a single hospital	65 % male,38.0 +/- 4.4 at time of injury, race not specified	I: <80 yrs old treated for compartment sydrome betwee '99-'04 E: other injuries that could cause impaired strength or motion, amputation, psychiatric disorder, disabled pts., those living >80 miles away

APPENDIX E, EVIDENCE TABLE 1. Studies on patient factors associated with polytrauma outcomes (Key Question 4)

Author, Year (ref.)	N enrolled, Tx v. controls	Exposure of interest	Control group: Comparator to exposure of interest	Pain-related outcomes measured	Timing of Outcomes	Is pain outcome a **main** outcome in
Vles, 2005(31)	N elegible =295; N enrolled=166	written questionnaire or a telephone interview	general population	EQ-5D-pain and discomfort scale Glasgow Outcome Scale and return to work status	1 yr post injury	No
Dougherty, 1999(32)	23 cases and 145 age and gender-matched controls from a national registry	none	none	SF-36 scores (including bodily pain)	given questionaire 27.5 years (on avg.) after surgery	Yes
Dougherty, 2001(33)	N = 72 total Group 1, n=28 Group 2, n=44	n/a	none	SF-36 scores (including bodily pain)	27.5 years (on avg.) after surgery	Yes, is one of several QOL indicators examined
Frink, 2007(34)	N=26	none--all had compartment syndrome treated by fasciotomy	none	reports of pain	2.4 years after hospital admission (on avg.)	No

APPENDIX E, EVIDENCE TABLE 1. Studies on patient factors associated with polytrauma outcomes (Key Question 4)

Author, Year (ref.)	Are results stratified or adjusted for polytrauma	Analytic method	Variables adjusted for in analysis or stratification
Vles, 2005(31)	not stratified but one of the determinants is number of inured body parts (one, two, two or more)	outcomes of eq-5d dichotomized to no problems/problems and tested by pearson chi-squared test. Index scores were compared using the Mann Whitness test for comparing two groups and Kruskal_Wallis test for ordered groups. Multivariable analyses were performed to evaluate joint effects on outcomes.	None
Dougherty, 1999(32)	No	bivariate comparisons	None
Dougherty, 2001(33)	Yes	bivariate comparisons	None
Frink, 2007(34)	Yes	bivariate comparisons	None

APPENDIX E, EVIDENCE TABLE 1. Studies on patient factors associated with polytrauma outcomes (Key Question 4)

Author, Year (ref.)	Results	Quality rating
Vles, 2005(31)	Factors associated the pain or discomfort dimension of the 5Q-5D are: ISS>=25 (p=<0.05); gender=female (p=<0.05); Injury to the chest or thoracic contents (p=<0.01); Injury to remaining body areas (not head, abdomen, chest, spine or extremity) (p=<0.01).	Fair
Dougherty, 1999(32)	Amputation smple scored lower on the physical functioning scale of the SF-36. Comparisons on the other 7 subscales revealed no significant differences. A third of sample continued to use prosthetics(25 + yrs. Post-injury)	Poor
Dougherty, 2001(33)	Polytrauma group scored significently lower on a measure of QOL compared w. a control group. ----polytrauma was not directly compared to single trauma	Fair to poor
Frink, 2007(34)	Compartment syndrome treated by fasciotomy led to impaired isokinetic muscle strenght of the injured leg. No diff. Though compairing polytrauma pts. To single trauma.	Fair

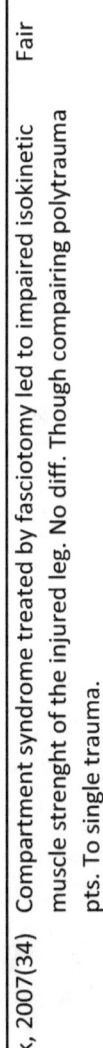

APPENDIX E, EVIDENCE TABLE 1. Studies on patient factors associated with polytrauma outcomes (Key Question 4)

Author, Year (ref.)	Title	Topic area	Study Design	Sample: All polytrauma patients, majority, or just included?	Aims
Lacoux, 2002(35)	Pain in traumatic upper limb amputees in Sierra Leone	Amputation, non-veteran	Cross sectional	Included	To study stump pain, phantom sensation, and phantom pain in 40 pts post-amputation.
Millstein, 1985(36)	A review of employment patterns of industrial amputees-- factors influencing rehabilitation	Amputation	Cross sectional	Included	The study investigated the current employment status of amputees and the factors that influenced successful return t work postamputation
Pezzin, 2000(37)	Rehabilitation and the long-term outcomes of persons with trauma-related amputations	Amputation, non-veteran	Cohort study, retrospective	Majority	To examine the long-term physical, social, and mental health outcomes of people who had trauma-related amputation. Also to explore factors affecting variation in outcomes and the role of inpatient rehab in improving vucntioning and well being.
Roganovic, 2006(38)	Pain syndromes after missile-caused peripheral nerve lesions: part 2---treatment	Peripheral nerve injury	Cohort study---retrospective	Included	To analyze treatment procedures and painful missle-caused nerve injuries and factors influencing the outcome

APPENDIX E, EVIDENCE TABLE 1. Studies on patient factors associated with polytrauma outcomes (Key Question 4)

Author, Year (ref.)	Setting	Sample demographics and other characteristics (include average time since injury at study baseline, if applicable)	Inclusion/exclusion criteria
Lacoux, 2002(35)	Study conducted in Sierra Leone - provides cross-cultural data	Non-veterans, Mean age 39.4 32 men, 8 women African	All amputees included, no exclusion criteria
Millstein, 1985(36)	amputee clinic at ontario worker compensation board	95% male, age 35, 12% multiple amputations	every person with amputation a result of work related accident between 1917 and 1981
Pezzin, 2000(37)	Pts who underwent trauma-related amputation at 1 specific hospital between '84-'94. They were then contacted and interviewed.	Non-VA, 87% male Mean age 32.9 (10.6)at time of injury. 75% white	Inclusion - discharged from hospital between '84-'94 following trauma-related amputation. Exclusion: amputation for non-injury reasons (e.g. diabetes), spinal cord injury or TBI
Roganovic, 2006(38)	single hospital in Serbia	not specified (not US patients) 90.5% male	pain syndromes related to missle trauma inclusion:nerve injury-related mechanism of pain, injury to missle, need for surgical apin treatment, and/or constant meds for >10 days exclusion : pain not related to missle-caused nerve injury

APPENDIX E, EVIDENCE TABLE 1. Studies on patient factors associated with polytrauma outcomes (Key Question 4)

Author, Year (ref.)	N enrolled, Tx v. controls	Exposure of interest	Control group: Comparator to exposure of interest	Pain-related outcomes measured	Timing of Outcomes	Is pain outcome a main outcome in
Lacoux, 2002(35)	N=40	n/a	n/a	Self-reports of pain	10-48 months after injury	Yes
Millstein, 1985(36)	1010pts total (117 with multiple amputations)	n/a	n/a	presence of stump and phantom/limb pain	variable	No
Pezzin, 2000(37)	N-78	n/a	Compared their sample trauma pts to mean population scores on the SF-36.	Quality of life scores	Average of 7.5 yrs after hospital discharge	Yes
Roganovic, 2006(38)	326	treatment differed based on type of injury	none	pain syndromes, pain intensity	varied based on procedure coducted ---at least one year	yes

APPENDIX E, EVIDENCE TABLE 1. Studies on patient factors associated with polytrauma outcomes (Key Question 4)

Author, Year (ref.)	Are results stratified or adjusted for polytrauma	Analytic method	Variables adjusted for in analysis or stratification
Lacoux, 2002(35)	Yes	bivariate comparisons	None
Millstein, 1985(36)	yes- by multiple vs. single amputation	bivariate comparisons	Not specified
Pezzin, 2000(37)	No	Mostly descriptive stats & logistic regression	None
Roganovic, 2006(38)	No	univariate and multivariate stats	None

APPENDIX E, EVIDENCE TABLE 1. Studies on patient factors associated with polytrauma outcomes (Key Question 4)

Author, Year (ref.)	Results	Quality rating
Lacoux, 2002(35)	All pts (100%) had stump pain. 93% had phantom sensations, but phantom pain was less common (33% unilateral vs. 18% bilateral)	Poor
Millstein, 1985(36)	When the influence of stump and phantom limb pain was examined, the data revealed that there was a high incidence of both kinds of pain. Their incidence was reported by 63% of upper limb amputees, 74 % of lower limb ammputees and 73% of multiple level amputees. Stump and phantom limb pain were identified as variables that were negatively associated wtih successful employment as subjects reporting higher levels of pain were less likely to be working.	Poor
Pezzin, 2000(37)	Trauma pts had poor QOL scores for physical functioning than the general population. No sig. Diff on mental health (7.5 yrs post-injury). 25% are sig. bothered by phantom pain. Nearly all pts. (97%) working at time of injury, but only 58% working at time of the study 0 and were working in less physically demanding positions. Several factors predicted whether pt. received inpt rehab tx (40% of pts): older at time of injury, +premorbid illness, non-white ethnicity, & pts who spent more days in the ICU at time of injury. Inpt rehab significantly improved health (QOL scores) & vocational prospects (more likely to return to work). White ethnicity had better outcomes than non-white.	Fair
Roganovic, 2006(38)	three factors predicted successful outcome: type o pain syndrome, severity of nerve injury, and absence of apin paroxysms rate of successful pain treatment differed based on pain diagnosis. Medications should be used to treat certain pain syndromes Adverse events: dizziness, nausea and /or headache(10%) in pateints treated with meds; 7.5% of pts after surgery.	Fair

APPENDIX E, EVIDENCE TABLE 1. Studies on patient factors associated with polytrauma outcomes (Key Question 4)

Author, Year (ref.)	Title	Topic area	Study Design	Sample: All polytrauma patients, majority, or just included?	Aims
Roganovic, 2006(39)	Pain syndromes after missle-caused peripheral nerve lesions: part 1—treatment	Complex regional, peripheral injury	Cohort study—retrospective	Included	to report on the clinical characteristics of pain and factors influencing pain intensity in pts. With missle-caused nerve injuries
Nampiaparampil, 2008(40)	Prevalence of Chronic Pain After traumatic Brain Injury	Headache, TBI	Systematic review	Included	To determine the prevalence of chronic pain as an underdiagnosed consequence of TBI and to review the interaction between chronic pain and severity of TBI as well as the characteristics of pain after T BI among civilians and combatants.
Ulvik, 2008(41)	Quality of life 2-7 years after major trauma	---	Cohort study—retrospective	All	To assess the potential impairmentin HRQol in trauma patients before injury and 2-7 years after discharge from the ICU. A further objective has been to study the following parameters a possible determinants of HRQOL: age, sex, time since trauma, Simplified Acute Physiology Score (SAPS) II, injury Severity Score (ISS), and severe head injury.
Stalp, 2002 (42)	Standardized Outcome Evaluation after Blunt Multiple Injuries by scoring Systems: A Clinical Follow-up Investigation 2 Years Injury	---	Cohort study—prospective	All	To evaluate the state of rehabilitation in patients with blunt multiple injuries 2 years after their initial injuries using several standardized scales.

APPENDIX E, EVIDENCE TABLE 1. Studies on patient factors associated with polytrauma outcomes (Key Question 4)

Author, Year (ref.)	Setting	Sample demographics and other characteristics (include average time since injury at study baseline, if applicable)	Inclusion/exclusion criteria
Roganovic, 2006(39)	single hospital in Serbia	veterans/active military ---not specified (not US patients) age range ,mean--12-63(mean=35.3 +/- 15, race not specified, 90% male	nerve injury--related mechanism od pain, injury two missle, need for surgical pain treatment, and/or constant meds. For >10 days
Nampiaparampil, 2008(40)	variable	variable-systematic review, all studies observational	Three studies that met all other criteria were excluded because they focused on individuals youger than 16 years.
Ulvik, 2008(41)	Norwegian 900 bed University hospital	81% male, average 39, mean ISS 25, 28% with sevre head injury , race-- not specified	Trauma pts admitted to ICU between 1998 and 2003 who completed flu in 2005
Stalp, 2002 (42)	multisite registry form 26 trauma centers in Germany	56% men, mean age=36, mean ISS=24, mean initial GCS=11	-- Blunt multiple injuries 2 years before follow-up investigation -- treated at level 1 trauma center

APPENDIX E, EVIDENCE TABLE 1. Studies on patient factors associated with polytrauma outcomes (Key Question 4)

Author, Year (ref.)	N enrolled, Tx v. controls	Exposure of interest	Control group: Comparator to exposure of interest	Pain-related outcomes measured	Timing of Outcomes	Is pain outcome a main outcome in
Roganovic, 2006(39)	326	different pts. Had different interventions depending on type of injury and pain syndrome	none	pain syndromes, pain intensity	days after surgery	yes
Nampiaparampil, 2008(40)	23 studies, 4206 total pts.	n/a	n/a	pain prevalence	variable	yes-pain prevalence
Ulvik, 2008(41)	210	n/a	n/a	EQ5D pain/discomfort	variable	No
Stalp, 2002 (42)	254	n/a	n/a	reports of pain	mean 2.2 yrs after injury	No

10/5/2010

APPENDIX E, EVIDENCE TABLE 1. Studies on patient factors associated with polytrauma outcomes (Key Question 4)

Author, Year (ref.)	Are results stratified or adjusted for polytrauma	Analytic method	Variables adjusted for in analysis or stratification
Roganovic, 2006(39)	No	univariate and multivariate stats ANOVA, kruskal-Walli, logistic regression	None
Nampiaparampil, 2008(40)	yes-severity of TBI	pooling data by adding across studies;bivariate anlyses	---
Ulvik, 2008(41)	yes-- by injury severity scores	multivariable regression	Age, sex, years since trauma, injury severity variables
Stalp, 2002 (42)	No	Bivariate comparisons only	None

APPENDIX E, EVIDENCE TABLE 1. Studies on patient factors associated with polytrauma outcomes (Key Question 4)

Author, Year (ref.)	Results	Quality rating
Roganovic, 2006(39)	Pain syndromes caused by missles differ significantly regarding time of pain onset, pain characteristics and other symptoms. Type of pain syndrome, multiple nerve damage, and early onset of pain areindependent predictors of intial pain intensity.	Fair
Nampiaparampil, 2008(40)	Twelve studies assessed headache apin in 1670 patients. Of these , 966 complained of chronic headache, yielding a prevalence of 57.8% (95% confidence interval [CI] 55.5%-60.2%). Among civilians, the prevalence of chronic pain was greater in patients with mild TBI (73.% [95%CI, 72.7%-77.9%])compared with moderate or severe TBI(32.1%[95%CI, 29.3%-34.9%]). twenty studies including 3289 civilian patients withTBI yielded a chronic pain prevalence of 51.5%(95% CI,49.8%-53.2%) . Three studies assessed TBI among 917 verterans and yielded a pain prevalence of 43.1%(95%CI, 39.9%-46.3%). PTSD may mediate chronic pain, but brain injury appears to have an independent correlation with chronic pain.	Fair
Ulvik, 2008(41)	--pts without severe head injury reported more problems with pain/discomfort -- years since trauma negatively associated with pain/ discomfort(p=0.035)	---
Stalp, 2002 (42)	In patients who reported restrictions of the lower extremity of. 52% indicated pain or impaired ability to walk caused by the injury to the foot and ankle, 31% to the kneee or thigh, and 17% to the femur or hip.	Fair

References in Evidence Table 1

1   Bay E, Donders J. Risk factors for depressive symptoms after mild-to-moderate traumatic brain injury. Brain Inj 2008;22(3):233-41.

2   Beetar JT, Guilmette TJ, Sparadeo FR. Sleep and pain complaints in symptomatic traumatic brain injury and neurologic populations. Archives of Physical Medicine & Rehabilitation 1996;77(12):1298-302.

3   Brenner C. Post-traumatic headache. J Neurosurgery 1944;1:379--391.

4   Bryant RA, Marosszeky JE, Crooks J, Baguley IJ, Gurka JA. Interaction of posttraumatic stress disorder and chronic pain following traumatic brain injury. Journal of Head Trauma Rehabilitation 1999;14(6):588-94.

5   Bushnik T, Englander J, Wright J. The Experience of Fatigue in the First 2 Years After Moderate-to-Severe Traumatic Brain Injury: A Preliminary Report. The Journal of head trauma rehabilitation 2008;23(1):17-24.

6   Cantor JB, Ashman T, Gordon W, Ginsberg A, Engmann C, Egan M, et al. Fatigue after traumatic brain injury and its impact on participation and quality of life. The Journal of head trauma rehabilitation 2008;23(1):41-51.

7   Cosgrove JL, Vargo M, Reidy ME. A prospective study of peripheral nerve lesions occurring in traumatic brain-injured patients. American Journal of Physical Medicine & Rehabilitation 1989;68(1):15-7.

8   Dawson DR, Schwartz ML, Winocur G, Stuss DT. Return to productivity following traumatic brain injury: cognitive, psychological, physical, spiritual, and environmental correlates. Disability & Rehabilitation 2007;29(4):301-13.

9   Guttman E. Postcontusional Headache. Lancet 1943;1:10-12.

10 Hillier SL, Sharpe MH, Metzer J. Outcomes 5 years post-traumatic brain injury(with further reference to neurophysical impairment and disability). Brain Injury 1997;11(9):661-75.

11 Hoffman JM, Pagulayan KF, Zawaideh N, Dikmen S, Temkin N, Bell KR. Understanding pain after traumatic brain injury: impact on community participation. American Journal of Physical Medicine & Rehabilitation 2007;86(12):962-9.

12 Lippert-Gruner M, Maegele M, Haverkamp H, Klug N, Wedekind C. Health-related quality of life during the first year after severe brain trauma with and without polytrauma. Brain Inj 2007;21(5):451-5.

13 Masson F, Maurette P, Salmi LR, Dartigues JF, Vecsey J, Destaillats JM, et al. Prevalence of impairments 5 years after a head injury, and their relationship with disabilities and outcome. Brain Injury 1996;10(7):487-97.

14   Olver JH, Ponsford JL, Curran CA. Outcome following traumatic brain injury: a comparison between 2 and 5 years after injury. Brain Injury 1996;10(11):841-8.

15   Walker WC, Seel RT, Curtiss G, Warden DL. Headache after moderate and severe traumatic brain injury: a longitudinal analysis. Archives of Physical Medicine & Rehabilitation 2005;86(9):1793-800.

16   Brenneman FD, Katyal D, Boulanger BR, Tile M, Redelmeier DA. Long-term outcomes in open pelvic fractures. Journal of Trauma-Injury Infection & Critical Care 1997;42(5):773-7.

17   Hebert JS, Burnham RS. The effect of polytrauma in persons with traumatic spine injury. A prospective database of spine fractures. Spine 2000;25(1):55-60.

18   Tran T, Thordarson D. Functional outcome of multiply injured patients with associated foot injury. Foot & Ankle International 2002;23(4):340-3.

19   Turchin DC, Schemitsch EH, McKee MD, Waddell JP. Do foot injuries significantly affect the functional outcome of multiply injured patients? Journal of Orthopaedic Trauma 1999;13(1):1-4.

20   Urquhart DM, Williamson OD, Gabbe BJ, Cicuttini FM, Cameron PA, Richardson MD, et al. Outcomes of patients with orthopaedic trauma admitted to level 1 trauma centres. ANZ Journal of Surgery 2006;76(7):600-6.

21   Zelle BA, Brown SR, Panzica M, Lohse R, Sittaro NA, Krettek C, et al. The impact of injuries below the knee joint on the long-term functional outcome following polytrauma. Injury 2005;36(1):169-77.

22   Anke AG, Stanghelle JK, Finset A, Roaldsen KS, Pillgram-Larsen J, Fugl-Meyer AR. Long-term prevalence of impairments and disabilities after multiple trauma. Journal of Trauma-Injury Infection & Critical Care 1997;42(1):54-61.

23   Brenneman FD, Redelmeier DA, Boulanger BR, McLellan BA, Culhane JP. Long-term outcomes in blunt trauma: who goes back to work? J Trauma 1997;42(5):778-81.

24   Dimopoulou I, Anthi A, Mastora Z, Theodorakopoulou M, Konstandinidis A, Evangelou E, et al. Health-related quality of life and disability in survivors of multiple trauma one year after intensive care unit discharge. American Journal of Physical Medicine & Rehabilitation 2004;83(3):171-6.

25   Fitzharris M, Fildes B, Charlton J, Kossmann T. General health status and functional disability following injury in traffic crashes. Traffic Injury Prevention 2007;8(3):309-20.

26   Holtslag HR, van Beeck EF, Lindeman E, Leenen LPH. Determinants of long-term functional consequences after major trauma. Journal of Trauma-Injury Infection & Critical Care 2007;62(4):919-27.

27   MacKenzie EJ, Morris JA, Jr., Jurkovich GJ, Yasui Y, Cushing BM, Burgess AR, et al. Return to work following injury: the role of economic, social, and job-related factors. Am J Public Health 1998;88(11):1630-7.

28 Meerding WJ, Looman CW, Essink-Bot ML, Toet H, Mulder S, van Beeck EF. Distribution and determinants of health and work status in a comprehensive population of injury patients. J Trauma 2004;56(1):150-61.

29 Mkandawire NC, Boot DA, Braithwaite IJ, Patterson M. Musculoskeletal recovery 5 years after severe injury: long term problems are common. Injury 2002;33(2):111-5.

30 Soberg HL, Bautz-Holter E, Roise O, Finset A. Long-term multidimensional functional consequences of severe multiple injuries two years after trauma: a prospective longitudinal cohort study. Journal of Trauma-Injury Infection & Critical Care 2007;62(2):461-70.

31 Vles WJ, Steyerberg EW, Essink-Bot ML, van Beeck EF, Meeuwis JD, Leenen LP. Prevalence and determinants of disabilities and return to work after major trauma. J Trauma 2005;58(1):126-35.

32 Dougherty PJ. Long-term follow-up study of bilateral above-the-knee amputees from the Vietnam War. Journal of Bone & Joint Surgery - American Volume 1999;81(10):1384-90.

33 Dougherty PJ. Transtibial amputees from the Vietnam War. Twenty-eight-year follow-up. Journal of Bone & Joint Surgery - American Volume 2001;83-A(3):383-9.

34 Frink M, Klaus A-K, Kuther G, Probst C, Gosling T, Kobbe P, et al. Long term results of compartment syndrome of the lower limb in polytraumatised patients. Injury 2007;38(5):607-13.

35 Lacoux PA, Crombie IK, Macrae WA. Pain in traumatic upper limb amputees in Sierra Leone. Pain 2002;99(1-2):309-12.

36 Millstein S, Bain D, Hunter GA. A review of employment patterns of industrial amputees--factors influencing rehabilitation. Prosthetics & Orthotics International 1985;9(2):69-78.

37 Pezzin LE, Dillingham TR, MacKenzie EJ. Rehabilitation and the long-term outcomes of persons with trauma-related amputations. Archives of Physical Medicine & Rehabilitation 2000;81(3):292-300.

38 Roganovic Z, Mandic-Gajic G. Pain syndromes after missile-caused peripheral nerve lesions: part 2--treatment. Neurosurgery 2006;59(6):1238-49; discussion 1249-51.

39 Roganovic Z, Mandic-Gajic G. Pain syndromes after missile-caused peripheral nerve lesions: part 1--clinical characteristics. Neurosurgery 2006;59(6):1226-36; discussion 1236-7.

40 Nampiaparampil DE. Prevalence of chronic pain after traumatic brain injury: a systematic review. JAMA 2008;300(6):711-9.

41 Ulvik A, Kvale R, Wentzel-Larsen T, Flaatten H. Quality of life 2-7 years after major trauma. Acta Anaesthesiologica Scandinavica 2008;52(2):195-201.

42   Stalp M, Koch C, Ruchholtz S, Regel G, Panzica M, Krettek C, et al. Standardized outcome evaluation after blunt multiple injuries by scoring systems: a clinical follow-up investigation 2 years after injury. Journal of Trauma-Injury Infection & Critical Care 2002;52(6):1160-8.

APPENDIX E, EVIDENCE TABLE 2. Ongoing research on pain in patients with polytrauma

Principal Investigator	Project Title	Main objective(s) of project	Study characteristics
Afari, N.	Headaches in veterans returning from Iraq/Afghanistan: relation to trauma and combat-related injury	To determine the relationship between Post-Traumatic Stress Disorder (PTSD), TBI, self-report of headaches, and combat-related injury in Operation Endjuring Freedom (OEF) and Operation Iraqi Freedom (OIF) veterans.	Study design: Cross-sectional Population: 343 male and female veterans registering for care at the VA San Diego Healthcare System between April and October 2006 Exposures: Combat Exposure Scale, injury during combat, serious head injury, PTSD, depression, substance abuse Outcomes: Prevalence and odds ratios of headaches (tension, migraine, or both) Timing of assessment: Upon enrollment for member services
Bair, M.	Evaluation of Stepped CAre for Chronic Pain (ESCAPE)	To compare the effectiveness of a stepped care intervention vs. usual care in OIF/OEF veterans with chronic and disabling musculoskeletal pain and to evaluate the impact of this intervention on pain-related disability, pain severity, psychological distress, and secondary outcomes (work functioning, health-related QOL, self-efficacy to manage pain, negative pain beliefs and coping, & satisfaction with treatment).	Study design: RCT Population: 300 OIF/OEF veterans with chronic and disabling musculoskeletal pain of the spine or extremities Intervention: Stepped care approach: 1) 12wks analgesic plus self-management program 2) 12wks cognitive behavioral therapy Comparator: not specified Outcomes: pain-related disability, pain severity, psychological distress, and secondary outcomes (work functioning, health-related QOL, self-efficacy to manage pain, negative pain beliefs and coping, & satisfaction with treatment) Timing of outcome assessment: baseline, 3 mos, 6, mos, 9 mos
Brandt, C. and Haskell, S.	Women Veterans Cohort Study	Aim I. To assess health care utilization, costs, and satisfaction during the complete 2 year healthcare coverage after discharge from service among female and male OEF/OIF veterans. Aim II. To assess changes in healthcare utilization, costs and satisfaction after the 2-year complete healthcare coverage ends. Aim III. To compare the diagnosis and treatment of stress associated conditions during the 2-year complete healthcare coverage	Study design: prospective cohort based on survey data Population: OEF/OIF veterans recruited from 5 VA Medical Centers Exposure: during 2-yr complete health coverage after discharge Comparator: after the 2-yr coverage ends Survey of healthcare ustilization, cost, satisfaction post-discharge, before and after 2-yr health coverage Outcomes: healthcare utilization, cost, satisfaction, stress, and pain scores Timing of assessment: baseline and every 12 months for 3+ years

APPENDIX E, EVIDENCE TABLE 2. Ongoing research on pain in patients with polytrauma

Principal Investigator	Main outcome measures	Measures of other conditions	Project status
Afari, N.	Self-report of headaches (yes,no) Self-report of diagnosis of migraines, tension headaches, or both (Yes, No)	Davidson Trauma Scale (score >=40 indicates PTSD) Combat Exposure Scale Drug Abuse Screening Test (substance abuse >=2) Self-report two-item depression screener (Yes, No) Self-report of injury during combat (Yes, No) Self-report of serious head injury (Yes, No)	Completed but no data published yet.
Bair, M.	Roland Disability Scale; Graded Chronic Pain Scale SF-12 Bodily Pain scale; BPI Interference scale Pain Catastrophizing Scale; Pain Stages of Change Questionnaire (PSOCQ); 3-item pain-specific patient satisfaction scale; Arthritis Self-Efficacy Scale	Patient Health Questionnaire (PHQ-9) for depression; Mental Component Summary Score (MCS) derived from the SF-12; PHQ anxiety scale; PCL-17, from DSM III-R criteria for PTSD; Global Rating of Change will be used to assess overall clinical response Work and Health Interview; Medical Outcomes Study SF-12, provides both a Physical and Mental Component Summary score Patient Health Questionnaire somatic symptom severity scale (PHQ-15); Patient Health Questionnaire stressor scale	Protocol has started, some recruitment
Brandt, C. and Haskell, S.	Brief Pain Inventory; VR-12; Veterans Health Survey pain care satisfaction	Combat Exposure scale, PCL and Trauma Questionnaire (PTSD), PRIME-MD.	Awaiting confirmation of funding for additional sites. Hoping to start national data work and survey work at 2 sites 3/08.

APPENDIX E, EVIDENCE TABLE 2. Ongoing research on pain in patients with polytrauma

Principal Investigator	Project Title	Main objective(s) of project	Study characteristics
Clark, M.E.	Pain and Emotional Disorders in Veterans with and without Polytrauma	a) Describe the prevalence, types, and course of pain and psychiatric disorders among patients with and without polytraumatic injuries; b) Determine whether patients with polytrauma have unique pain-related or emotional problems compared to OEF and OIF returnees registered for VA care but without polytrauma; c) Identify risk factors for the development of chronic pain and emotional disorders in these cohorts; d) Determine the interaction of emotional disorder comorbidities with pain or emotional symptom severity; and e) Describe the functional outcomes, associated disabilities, and community reintegration challenges associated with pain and emotional disorders among OEF/OIF service members with and without polytrauma.	Study design: prospective cohort using structured interviews Population: OEF/OIF military personnel; cross-sectional samples of 150-200 polytrauma and 300-400 non-polytrauma OEF/OIF military personnel from two sites (Minneapolis and Tampa VAs) Exposure: Polytrauma patients Comparator: Veterans without polytrauma Outcomes: Prevalence of pain and psychiatric disorders; risk factors for the development of chronic pain and emotional disorders; effect of emotional disorder comorbidities on pain; functional outcomes and disabilities. Sub-studies will be used to validate a new measure of deployment stress exposure, assess VA pain and emotional treatment satisfaction, determine 12-month incidence of new-onset pain and mental health problems, and evaluate the frequency and type of non-VA medical service utilization among OEF/OIF medical care registrants. Timing of assessment: baseline, 6 mo, 12 months
Gallagher, R.	Regional Anesthesia Military Battlefield Pain Outcomes Study	1) Quantify and characterize short-term and long-term effects traumatic extremity injuries during combat on post-injury pain, health-related quality of life (HRQOl), functional status, social reintegration, psychological adjustment and substance abuse among returning Iraq/Afghanistan veterans 2) Evaluate the efficacy of early aggressive advanced regional anesthetic interventional techniques on neuropathic pain, HRQOL, and mental health disorders among soldiers at 2-yrs post-injury	Study design: prospective cohort study based on medical records and interviews Population: OEF/OIF soldiers with one or more maligned or amputated limbs Exposure: traumatic extremity injuries Intervention: early aggressive advanced regional anesthetic techniques Outcome: pain, health-related QOL, functional status, social reintegration, psychological adjustment, substance abuse Timing of outcome assessment: baseline and 2-yrs post injury
Gironda, R.J.	Chronic Headache among OEF/OIF Veterans Exposed to Blasts	The purpose of the current study is to provide an initial evaluation of the clinical characteristics and treatment of headache conditions among OEF/OIF veterans who have been exposed to blasts during deployment. Is brief cognitive-behavioral headache management treatment (BCBHMT) feasible and effective for the reduction of blast-related headache frequency and associated disability?	Study design: case series Population: OEF/OIF veterans referred to the JAHVH PRC Blast Injury Clinic (Tampa) Intervention: cognitive-behavioral headache management treatment (BCBHMT) Outcomes: changes in headache severity and duration, unctional disability, and health-related quality of life; PTSD symptoms; sleep problems; fatigue symptoms; Timing of outcome assessment: Baseline and 3 months

APPENDIX E, EVIDENCE TABLE 2. Ongoing research on pain in patients with polytrauma

Principal Investigator	Main outcome measures	Measures of other conditions	Project status
Clark, M.E.	Military Hx; Pain Hx; MH Hx; Pain Dx; Pain Intensity; Pain-related interference (POQ); CPCI; CPQ; FABQ; STAI; CES-D; sleep measure (SPQ); fatigue measure (MFSI-SF); relationship measure (DAS-SF).	Psychiatric Dx via structured interview (M.I.N.I.); VA PTSD screen; CAGE; Blast exposure; medical Dx; depression and anxiety as above.	Approved; funded; still waiting HSR&D disbursement of 1st-years funds.
Gallagher, R.	1) TOPS (Treatment Outcomes in Pain Survey) 2) BPI 3) Neuropathic Pain Scale 4) Behavioral Health Laboratory Inventory 5) Injury Severity Index 6) Post-discharge treatment	Depression, PTSD, Substance Abuse	In progress
Gironda, R.J.	McGill Pain Questionnaire; Headache Disability Index; CES-D; STAI- State scale; Multidimensional Fatigue Symptom Inventory (Short Form); Sleep Problems Questionnaire; PTSD Symptoms Checklist Military Version; RBANS	CES-D; STAI- State scale; Multidimensional Fatigue Symptom Inventory (Short Form); Sleep Problems Questionnaire; PTSD Symptoms Checklist Military Version; RBANS	Recruitment has begun.

APPENDIX E, EVIDENCE TABLE 2. Ongoing research on pain in patients with polytrauma

Principal Investigator	Project Title	Main objective(s) of project	Study characteristics
Helmer, D.	Pain, mental health, and daily function in OIF/OEF veterans	To describe the pain concerns of OIF/OEF veterans, examine the association between pain and comorbid mental health concerns, and model the impact of these concerns on daily functioning.	Study design: cross-sectional, retrospective review of self-administered clinical intake/screening data Population: The first 233 OIF/OEF veterans with complete data evaluated at the War-Related Illness and Injury Study Center (WRIISC) in East Orange, NJ (June 2005-August 2007) Outcomes: Pain, mental health comorbidity, daily functioning Timing of outcome assessment: at time of clinical intake/screening
Kerns, R.	Pain Assessment in Polytrauma Rehabilitation Centers (PRCs)	Evaluate usability and utility of CPRS pain assessment templates in two PRC sites, modify education materials in support of these templates, and develop and pilot pain reports for clinicians based on these templates. Secondary objectives are to develop a pain assessment database and identify best practices for pain care in this patient population.	Study design: Qualitative and quantitative information collected from clinicians two PRCs (Minneapolis and Tampa). Population: Providers and nursing staff in two PRCs (Minneapolis and Tampa). Intervention: The pain template contains modules designed for initial comprehensive assessment and reassessment of pain. Outcomes: Pain intensity, pain quality, pain location, alleviating and aggravating factors, medication use, and pain-related disability including mood, sleep, physical activity, sleep and work Timing of outcome assessment: Physicians and nurses are encouraged to comprehensively assess all new patients when they present to the PRC.
Lawrence, V.A.	Long-term Outcomes in Burned OEF/OIF Veterans (LOBO)	To assess long term outcomes in OEF/OIF veterans with combat burn injury, combat nonburn injury, and in a 3rd cohort of civilian burn patients	Study design: Prospective cohort Population: OEF/OIF veterans with a combat burn injury, combat nonburn injury, and civilian burn patients Exposure groups: burn injury, non-burn injury; combat veterans, civilians Outcomes: PTSD, depression, sleep Timing of outcome assessment: Baseline, 1, 2, 3, and 4 years.
Lew, H.	Characterization and Care Coordination of Polytrauma Patients	To study & describe characteristics of polytrauma patients, including the nature and severity of cognitive, emotional, physical and overall functional impairment.	Study design: Cross-sectional Population: OIF/OEF patients injured by explosive devices or blasts Exposure groups: blast injury alone; blast TBI; non-blast TBI; PTSD; non-PTSD Outcomes: nature and severity of cognitive, emotional, physical and overall functional impairment. Timing of outcome assessment: clinic visit
Lew, H.	Clinical Characteristics of Patients with Polytrauma and Blast-Related Injuries	To describe the clinical characteristics, interventions and outcomes for inpatients with polytrauma and blast-related injuries treated through the Polytrauma Rehabilitation Center (PRC) at the VAPAHCS.	Study design: retrospective review of routine care data Population: veterans who were inpatients at the 4 PRCs. Exposure: polytrauma and blast-related injuries Outcomes: clinical characteristics, interventions; sleep disturbances, post-concussive symptoms, combat-related stress, functional independence

VA-ESP Pain in Polytrauma

10/5/2010

APPENDIX E, EVIDENCE TABLE 2. Ongoing research on pain in patients with polytrauma

Principal Investigator	Main outcome measures	Measures of other conditions	Project status
Helmer, D.	Veterans RAND (VR)-36 Bodily Pain (BP) and Role Physical (RP) scales; chronic widespread pain (CWP)	1) Patient Health Questionnaire (PHQ) 2) Post-traumatic stress disorder (PTSD), depression, and problem alcohol use screening instruments (AUDIC-C).	Completed but no data published yet.
Kerns, R.	Measures included in the templates themselves which are pain intensity (NRS 0-10 scale , pain quality, pain location, alleviating and aggravating factors, medication use, and pain-related disability including mood, sleep, physical activity, sleep and work.	The pain template contains a module designed to assist clinicians in evaluating pain in patients with cognitive impairment. The template does not explicitly collect data regarding the nature or magnitude of the impairment, but does provide support for collecting accurate pain assessments in the context of cognitive impairment.	The project has been approved and is in progress.
Lawrence, V.A.	McGill Pain Questionnaire – Short Form SF-12	PCL-C and M (PTSD), CES-D (Depression), Epworth sleepiness scale. AUDIT-C	In progress
Lew, H.	VAS	PTSD (PCL) Memory Loss/Cognition (Neuropsych measures)	in progress.
Lew, H.	Per medical record	Sleep disturbances, post-concussive sx, combat-related stress, FIM	Ongoing—some preliminary findings

APPENDIX E, EVIDENCE TABLE 2. Ongoing research on pain in patients with polytrauma

Principal Investigator	Project Title	Main objective(s) of project	Study characteristics
Lew, H.	Predicting Rehabilitation Costs for VA Patients with Traumatic Brain Injury	To estimate cost of care for a sample of TBI patients. Objectives include: 1) To determine differences, if any, in cost patterns for rehabilitation among OEF/OIF returnees with combat-related TBI versus those with non-combat related TBI 2) To compare the utility of Life Care Planning and FIM scores in predicting total rehabilitation costs fro the same period. 3) To examine how PTSD impacts future outcomes and costs associated with combat-related TBI.	Study design: retrospective cohort study Population: a sample of OEF/OIF patients with TBI, physical injury, and emotional trauma, discharged from the PRC, and treated at the Palo Alto and Tampa VA Exposure groups: Combat-related TBI, non-combat TBI; PTSD Outcomes: Cost of care for rehabilitation; utility of Life Care Planning and FIM scores for predicting cost of care Timing of outcome assessment: Up to 12 months after initial discharge
Roy M.J.	The ViRTICo Trial: Virtual Reality Therapy & Imaging in Combat Veterans	1. Distinguish between four groups of 22 GWOT veterans each, those with: PTSD and TBI combined; PTSD alone; TBI alone; and neither PTSD nor TBI, using an Affective Stroop test as well as digital photographs taken in Iraq and Afghanistan, in conjunction with functional magnetic resonance imaging (fMRI). 2. Demonstrate that VRET is non-inferior to the current first-line therapy for which there is best evidence, Prolonged Exposure (PE), in the treatment of OIF/OEF combat veterans with PTSD.	Study design: controlled clinical trial Population: Global War on Terror (GWOT) veterans with PTSD and TBI combined; PTSD alone; TBI alone; and neither PTSD nor TBI. Intervention: Virtual Reality Exposure Therapy & Imaging Comparator: Prolonged exposure (current first-line therapy). Outcomes: functional health and disability - 6 domains: understanding and communicating, getting around, self care, getting along with others, household and work activities, participation in society Timing of outcome assessment: Baseline (following assessment at Walter Reed); post-treatment; 12-week follow up
Siddharthan, K.	Telerehabilitation of OEF/OIF combat wounded with TBI	To provide for care coordination and monitor functional and cognitive outcomes of 45 veterans treated and discharged from the James Haley Veterans Hospital in Tampa, FL with combat related TBI	Study design: cohort Population: Veterans with combat related TBI Exposure: Pain medications Outcomes: Adverse effects of pain medication on functional and cognitive outcomes (withdrawal symptoms/suicidal tendencies/addiction/accidents, etc.)
Storzbach, DM	Multidiscipline Assessment of Blast Victims for Cognitive Rehabilitation	To determine whether blast exposure during military service is associated with increased risk for neuropsychological deficits and/or psychiatric disorder, and to determine whether blast-related symptoms of post-concussive syndrome are caused by the psychiatric effects of the wartime environment, neuropsychological effects of traumatic brain injury, or sub-optimal motivation.	Study design: prospective cohort Population: OEF/OIF veterans in one of 3 exposure groups Exposure groups: 1) explosion-exposed and reports <= 0.5 hour loss of consciousness, or <=24 post-traumatic amnesia following the explosion(s); 2) explosion-exposed without subsequent symptoms of concussions; 3) Unexposed to explosions Outcomes: neuropsychological deficits and psychiatric disorder Timing of outcome assessment: 1 assessment visit; 1st participant enrolled 4/29/08, expected to continue at least through 8/09.

APPENDIX E, EVIDENCE TABLE 2. Ongoing research on pain in patients with polytrauma

Principal Investigator	Main outcome measures	Measures of other conditions	Project status
Lew, H.	Functional Independence Measure: VAS	PTSD (PCL), Costs, Cognitive status (neuropsych data)	Ongoing
Roy M.J.	SF-36 World Health Organization Disability Assessment Schedule – II (WHODAS-II)	The primary outcome measure for judging success will be a 30% reduction in CAPS score at the end of treatment. Additional outcome measures will include a 30% reduction in CAPS scores at the end of a 12-week follow up period, significant reductions in scores on measures of other psychiatric disorders such as anxiety and depression, and a significant reduction in associated functional impairment at these endpoints on the SF-36 and WHODAS-II.	In progress
Siddharthan, K.	FIM/FAM and CHART for community Integration	Effects of drug therapy for pain management on cognitive deficits and mental health.	In progress
Storzbach, DM	Pittsburgh Sleep Quality Index (PSQI; Buysse et al., 1989); • British Columbia Post Concussive Symptom Inventory (BC-PSI; Iverson, 2005); Ruff Neurobehavioral Inventory: Cognition, Pain, Work Questionnaire (RNBI: CPW; Ruff & Hibbard, 2003); Test of Memory Malingering (TOMM; Tombaugh, 1996); PTSD Checklist; Military Version (PCL - M; Weathers & Ford, 1996); Personality Assessment Inventory (PAI; Morey, 1991)	Ruff Neurobehavioral Inventory: Cognition and Work Questionnaire (RNBI: CPW)	In progress

APPENDIX E, EVIDENCE TABLE 2. Ongoing research on pain in patients with polytrauma

Principal Investigator	Project Title	Main objective(s) of project	Study characteristics
Walker, R.L.	Evaluation of Polytrauma Pain	The primary objective of this study is to retrospectively examine the pain experiences of those soldiers and veterans who have incurred polytraumatic injuries during Operation Iraqi Freedom/Operation Enduring Freedom (OIF/OEF) conflicts.	Study design: retrospective chart review Population: OIF/OEF veterans with polytrauma injuries and were treated at the JAHVH-PRC between 2003-2006. Exposures: Nature, extent, and treatment of polytrauma injuries (on admission) Outcomes: Previous pain treatment (before admission); level of cognitive functioning (at admission and discharge); pain intensity scores (at admission and discharge); diagnose(s); pain location(s) (at admission and discharge); pain duration; pain management/interventions utilized during rehabilitation; pain management consult(s) initiated; co-morbid emotional symptoms and treatments provided Timing of outcome assessment: indicated in outcomes, above
Walker, W.	Concurrent Validity of Four Pain Intensity Scales in persons with Polytrauma and Cognitive Impairment	A preliminary analysis to examine the concurrent validity of four pain intensity scales in the traumatic brain injury (TBI) inpatient rehabilitation population.	Study design: prospective randomized measurement study Population: 15 consecutive adult patients who were admitted for acute rehabilitation within 12 months of major trauma, who reported pain initially, and consented to participate Interventions: pain assessment; memory assessment Outcomes: Current pain on days 0, 3, 7, 10, & 14; vividly remembered "worst pain ever" on Day 0 and 14 Timing of outcome assessment: Days 0, 3, 7, 10, & 14
Widerstrom-Noga, E.	Validity and reliability of proton magnetic resonance spectroscopy as a diagnostic and outcome measure in clinical pain trials involving people with spinal cord injury.	The present study will determine the validity and reliability of Magnetic Resonance Spectroscopy (MRS) as a diagnostic and outcome measure for clinical trials involving SCI chronic pain populations. The long-term goal of our pain research is to improve the management of chronic neuropathic pain following SCI.	Study design: measurement study Population: 60 persons with SCI and chronic neuropathic pain, 25 persons with SCI without neuropathic pain, and 25 able-bodied control subjects Intervention: Magnetic Resonance Spectroscopy (MRS) Outcomes: Pain, functioning, and mood; neurological examinations and MRS imaging procedures Timing of outcome assessment: 2-4 weeks after 1st session (baseline screening); additionally, 2-4 weeks after 1st session for SCI patients with neuropathic pain.

APPENDIX E, EVIDENCE TABLE 2. Ongoing research on pain in patients with polytrauma

Principal Investigator	Main outcome measures	Measures of other conditions	Project status
Walker, R.L.	Per medical record	The only measure of cognitive functioning that was collected in this study was the patients' Rancho score that was assigned by the treating team upon admission and discharge. Data regarding psychological diagnoses was collected, along with information on what type of psychological (or psychiatric) treatment was conducted during rehabilitation.	The data has been collected for this project, but only portions of the data have been published up to this point in time.
Walker, W.	Faces pain scale, verbal descriptor scale (VDS), color analogue scale (CAS) and numerical (0-10) box-scale (BS-11)	Memory Orientation & Amnesia Test	In progress. As of March 13, "The study is ongoing with a recruitment goal of 60 subjects."
Widerstrom-Noga, E.	Medical History and Demographic questionnaire Pain History Form Multidimensional Pain Inventory (MPI) Numerical Rating Scales (NRS)	Functional Independence Measure (FIM) Craig Handicap Assessment and Reporting Technique (CHART) Spielberger State-Trait Anxiety Inventory (STAI) Coping Strategies Questionnaire (CSQ) Beck Depression Inventory (BDI) Structured interview to rule out major psychiatric illness and major depression Folstein Mini-Mental Status Examination to screen out traumatic brain injury	Ongoing

www.ingramcontent.com/pod-product-compliance
Lightning Source LLC
Chambersburg PA
CBHW081449170526
45166CB00008B/2363